The Guide to Living with Bladder Cancer

The Guide to Living with Bladder Cancer

Mark P. Schoenberg, M.D., F.A.C.S.
*and the Faculty and Staff of the Johns Hopkins
Genitourinary Oncology Group*

The Johns Hopkins University Press
Baltimore and London

M.P.S. dedicates this book to R.J.A.

© 2000 The Johns Hopkins University Press
All rights reserved. Published 2000
Printed in the United States of America on acid-free paper
9 8 7 6 5 4 3 2 1

The Johns Hopkins University Press
2715 North Charles Street
Baltimore, Maryland 21218–4363
www.press.jhu.edu

Illustrations by Jacqueline Schaffer.

Library of Congress Cataloging-in-Publication Data will be found at the end of this book.
A catalog record for this book is available from the British Library.

ISBN 0-8018-6405-4
ISBN 0-8018-6406-2 (pbk.)

CONTENTS

CONTRIBUTORS

Mark P. Schoenberg, M.D., F.A.C.S., Associate Professor, Department of Urology and Oncology, the Johns Hopkins University School of Medicine

David A. Bluemke, M.D., Ph.D., Associate Professor of Radiology, Director of MR Imaging, Department of Radiology, the Johns Hopkins University School of Medicine

Michael A. Carducci, M.D., Assistant Professor of Oncology, the Johns Hopkins University School of Medicine

Angelo M. DeMarzo, M.D., Ph.D., Instructor, Department of Pathology, the Johns Hopkins University School of Medicine

Theodore L. DeWeese, M.D., Assistant Professor of Radiation Oncology, the Johns Hopkins University School of Medicine

Mario L. Eisenberger, M.D., Professor of Oncology and Urology, the Johns Hopkins University School of Medicine and the James Buchanan Brady Department of Urology

Srinivas Mandavili, M.D., Fellow, Department of Pathology, the Johns Hopkins University School of Medicine

Dorothy L. Rosenthal, M.D., Professor of Pathology, Oncology, and Gynecology and Obstetrics and Director of Cytopathology, the Johns Hopkins University School of Medicine

Victoria J. W. Sinibaldi, R.N.-C., M.S., C.A.N.P., the Johns Hopkins Oncology Center

Joanne M. Walker, R.N., M.S., C.E.N.T., Department of Surgical Nursing, Enterostomal Therapy, the Johns Hopkins Hospital

Jenifer Willmann, M.D., Resident, Department of Radiology, the Johns Hopkins University School of Medicine

Marcia Wills, M.D., Fellow, Department of Pathology, the Johns Hopkins University School of Medicine

INTRODUCTION

Bladder cancer is the fourth most common cancer among American men and the eighth most common cancer among American women. Many people who have bladder cancer become very knowledgeable about the disease, but otherwise bladder cancer is a type of cancer about which most people know very little.

Being diagnosed with any kind of cancer can be very frightening. If you or a loved one is diagnosed with bladder cancer, the first thought that may come into your head is that this is a fatal disease and your or your loved one's days are numbered. Most people, when learning for the first time that they have cancer of any type, hear only the word *cancer* and nothing else. When the doctor first tells a person that he or she has cancer, the person, understandably, may stop listening and start focusing on his or her own worst fears. It may take several more conversations—with doctors, nurses, and other health care professionals, as well as with family members and friends—before the diagnosis starts to come into focus and the person can begin to cope.

Once things have settled down and the diagnosis has been placed in some perspective, the patient and his or her family and friends start to take an interest in research and information-gathering about the health problem that has been diagnosed. Once their diagnosis has been circulated among concerned family members and close friends, many patients begin receiving calls from all over, even from second cousins of ex-spouses, offering recommendations for surgeons, therapeutic programs, herbal remedies, and so on. It is the nature of people to take an interest in one another, and many patients are greatly helped by the interest, efforts, and research of family members and friends. Sometimes, however, the diagnosis of a potentially serious illness elicits more help and advice than the patient or family can possibly put to immediate or good use. One of the biggest problems people face is sifting through all of the available information to make a rational decision at a time of personal crisis and upheaval.

This is particularly true now, in the information age. The personal computer has brought the National Medical Library and the Internet, with its various forums and chat groups, into every computer owner's home. This is both a blessing and a curse for many patients and their families. The electronic world is full of information—much of it useful, some of it not. It can be difficult to make the distinction, especially at a time when your emotions are unsteady and you may be vulnerable. We used to follow a particular Internet cancer forum but stopped dropping in after we became convinced that the information being traded was primarily anecdotal, not based on scientific evidence, and frequently misleading. That experience is one reason we wrote this book. We also wanted to respond to requests by the many patients who have asked for an accessible summary for the lay consumer of what's known about bladder cancer and its treatments.

As you will learn in the following pages, bladder cancer is not one disease. From what is currently known, it is reasonably clear that bladder cancer is at least two different illnesses, one that is usually nonaggressive and relatively easy to control and another that is aggressive and can require extensive therapy. But while bladder cancer is a potentially serious health problem, it is not an emergency, even in its most dangerous forms.

In treating patients with cancer, we have found that many people want to act right away. With the new diagnosis of disease hanging over their heads, they think that to keep the cancer from spreading surgery must be done soon—even as soon as the day after diagnosis. What is probably more important than immediate action is being well informed about different therapies and their track records. *What* you do, in this case, is usually more important than when you do it.

Many lay people become knowledgeable about a disease once it affects them personally, but people are very different in terms of how much they want to know. Some want to know all the details of current scientific research on the disease, while others simply want to know when their problem is going to be fixed so they can get back to their families and their normal lives. Most people want something in between.

We also know that gathering information about medical therapy can be frustrating and time-consuming. In addition, you may get a fair amount of conflicting advice about some issues and virtually complete agreement from different doctors about other aspects of your care.

We have written this book for people with bladder cancer and their families, with the idea that they will read what they want—and need—and skip the rest. In your reading, you may want to skip around from chapter to chapter, because some material will apply to you and other material will not be relevant to your situation. Some chapters apply to both kinds of bladder cancer, others apply to one kind or the other.

Doctors often find that some patients feel guilty when they or a loved one becomes ill. Patients will ask if they have done something to bring the disease on themselves. Many men and women with cancer look back on their lives and ask themselves and their doctors what they did to get cancer. The answer for most patients—and certainly for the majority of bladder cancer patients—is that doctors don't know what causes disease. Some forms of environmental cancer-causing substances and chemicals, such as components of cigarette smoke, are known to contribute to the development of bladder tumors. However, many of our patients don't smoke and have never smoked, so smoking is not the only problem.

Another worry of most patients who are parents is the concern that their children and possibly grandchildren will develop bladder cancer because "cancer genes" run in the family. Luckily, bladder cancer does not tend to run in families. (More information about this topic appears later in this book.)

Some of our patients are very interested in the cancer-preventing properties of certain foods and herbal remedies. One, in particular, likes to send us information from various sources about new plants and nutritional additives that may decrease the likelihood of recurrence of bladder cancer. We want to be completely candid about this topic at the outset so that you won't read the whole book and be disappointed at the end. The fact is, very little is known about the effect of diet on the development of bladder cancer. Almost nothing is known about the impact of changing your diet after a diagnosis of bladder cancer, on the chance that the disease will respond more favorably either to conventional or alternative therapies that you will read about later in the book. Accordingly, this book contains very little information about foods, herbs, and homeopathic treatments for bladder cancer. That is not because all of these therapies and approaches lack merit; so far, however, they remain unproved. Perhaps as research on truly "alternative" therapies progresses, we'll be able to say more in the future about these approaches.

A few words about the range of health care providers involved in helping people with bladder cancer. The treatment of bladder cancer draws upon the skills, expertise, and talents of professionals from many disciplines, including medical and radiation oncology, pathology, radiology, and special branches of nursing, including oncologic nursing and enterostomal therapy. (See list below for more information about these specialists.) Bladder cancer is frequently diagnosed and initially treated by urologists. Urologists are physicians who specialize in the surgical and medical management of diseases of the urinary tract and male reproductive organs.

Health care professionals involved in the care of bladder cancer patients include the following:

Urologist: A trained surgeon specializing in the treatment of diseases of the urinary tract

Medical Oncologist: A physician trained in the medicinal treatment of cancers

Radiation Oncologist: A physical trained in the use of high-energy technologies such as x-rays to treat cancers

Radiologist: A physician trained in the diagnostic use of imaging technologies such as CT, ultrasound & MR

Pathologist: A physician trained in the microscopic analysis of tissues

Cytopathologist: A physician trained in microscopic techniques to analyze cells obtained from a variety of sources such as urine

Enterostomal therapist: A nurse trained in the specialized care of patients with stomas or ostomies

Oncology nurse specialist: A nurse trained in the specialized care of patients receiving treatment for cancer, such as chemotherapy

There is almost always more than one way to achieve a desired goal in medicine, so one objective of this book is to introduce you to various forms of bladder cancer therapy. Although it is not possible to describe the management of every clinical situation, in this book we try to explain how we approach the evaluation and treatment of the commoner types of bladder cancer and the problems caused by these tumors and their treatments.

This book is the work of a group of people who get together each week to determine how best to treat patients with bladder cancer. One of the most important aspects of our interaction as professionals and as people is that we all recognize that no one person has all of the answers to the management of bladder cancer (or of most other medical problems). We work together not only because we like to but also, frankly, because we need to. We all took a part in writing this book and putting it together. We have integrated the material to make it read or sound like one person talking to you, but you may hear some different voices here and there, from chapter to chapter. We tell you this to emphasize that this is a team effort designed to take you logically from the initial discovery of a bladder tumor through the standard diagnostic evaluation of the problem, then to the treatment and into the recovery phase of this illness. Along the way, many of our patients rely upon the different skills of the people who helped put this book together.

Each contributor to this book has written about what he or she does as if the potential readers of the book were members of the family calling for advice about a medical problem. We have used medical terminology that you are likely to encounter and therefore need to understand, but we have also attempted to explain technical language so you do not need a background in health care to read this book. We have also asked our patients to participate in this book; their impressions and observations about their treatments and their life after bladder cancer are included throughout the book (in shaded boxes), and their suggestions are summarized in chapter 9.

The book is organized into nine chapters, which stand alone as descriptions of specific aspects of bladder cancer care:

—Chapter 1 describes the structure and function of the normal urinary tract and provides a "geography lesson" on the parts of the body you need to know about in order to understand the *how* and *why* of different therapies for bladder cancer.

—Chapter 2 provides an overview of bladder cancer and information about risk factors for bladder cancer.

—Chapter 3 describes symptoms of bladder cancer and introduces the tests used to discover and diagnose bladder tumors.

—Chapter 4 details how 75 percent of bladder tumors can be removed without ever making an incision in the skin.

—Chapter 5 describes the major surgery that some patients will need for the treatment of bladder cancer.

—Chapter 6 is devoted to issues related to the very important topic of life after surgery, including life with various forms of urinary tract reconstruction.

—Chapter 7 describes alternatives to surgery that can be used to preserve the bladder even if advanced cancer is discovered.

—Chapter 8 details the use of intravenous or "total body" chemotherapy for treatment of bladder tumors that have spread beyond the confines of the bladder itself.

—Chapter 9 passes along some advice from our patients that we thought you might find helpful.

No book will answer all of your questions. It is our hope that after reading this book, you will understand bladder cancer better and feel that you can actively participate in making decisions about the course of your treatment.

The Guide to Living with Bladder Cancer

CHAPTER ONE

Some Anatomical Geography

Let's get oriented. To understand anything about a disease process, you have to start with an understanding of where things are in your body and what is normal, just like medical students do during the first year of their studies. To understand how bladder cancer is treated and what the various treatment options mean to you, it helps to have a clear picture of the system of organs that make up the urinary tract, of which the bladder is a principal player.

People who have never seen the inside of a human body have different ideas about what it looks like. One common misconception is that the body is a bloody mess inside, and therefore surgery must be a gruesome business. Nothing could be further from the truth. The human body is exceptionally tidy, and the organs that sustain life are all beautifully designed, compact, and elegant. There is no sports car that is as well designed under the hood.

Let's get our bearings. Since the job of the urinary system is to filter blood and produce waste material (urine), it is convenient to think of the system in terms of water running downhill. The *kidneys* are the top of the urinary tract. They are located in the upper abdomen, lying just underneath the breathing muscle called the diaphragm, which is protected by the lower portion of the rib cage. The other components of the urinary tract we will talk about are the *ureters*, tubes that carry urine from the kidneys to the bladder; the *bladder* itself, a muscular, balloon-shaped organ that stores urine and then squeezes it out at the appropriate moment; and

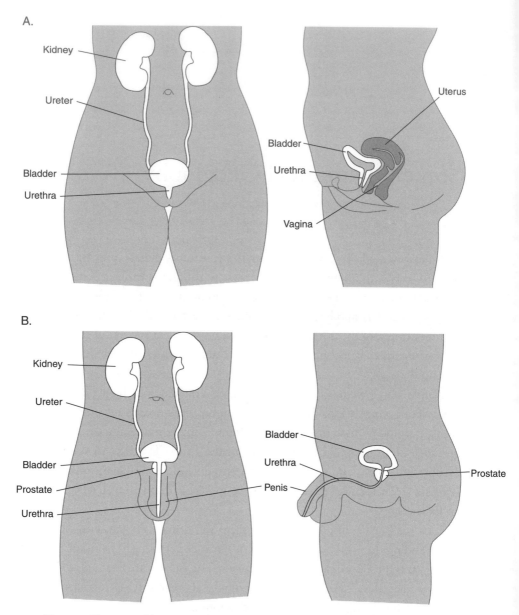

Kidney

Ureter

Bladder

Urethra

Uterus

Bladder

Urethra

Vagina

B.

Kidney

Ureter

Bladder

Prostate

Urethra

Bladder

Urethra

Penis

Prostate

Fig. 1.1. The normal location and structure of the upper and lower urinary tract in the female (A) and male (B).

the *urethra*, the tube that carries urine from the bladder to the outside of the body. There are other important organs in the area, such as the prostate in men and the vagina, uterus, and ovaries in women. Let's start our interior journey where the process begins.

The Kidneys

Urine, the principal but by no means only product of the urinary tract, is made by the kidneys, two bean-shaped organs that reside in the back of the upper abdomen, in the cavity that also contains the intestinal tract, liver, pancreas, and spleen. Unlike the digestive tract, most of which lies within a sack called the *peritoneum*, the kidneys and the rest of the urinary tract lie behind this thin protective covering and are thus referred to collectively as *retro* (behind) *peritoneal structures*.

The kidneys are amazingly hardworking organs. Packed full of blood vessels, they filter approximately 20 percent of the total body blood volume each minute. Each kidney, dark brown in color, weighs between ten and twenty ounces, depending on the size of the owner, and is approximately three by five by one inch in size. The kidneys act like factories processing a raw material (blood) that contains the by-products of digestion and normal bodily functions. They filter out the waste products and create a substance that can be easily eliminated, urine. The average 150-pound man excretes two quarts of urine a day.

Though paired, the two kidneys function individually. Each is a self-contained unit capable of doing all of the work of both if the need arises. Actually, the average adult can live a normal life with only about one half of one kidney, a lifesaving fact should one of the kidneys be damaged either by trauma or illness.

In addition to their waste-processing functions, the kidneys also play an important role in the control of blood pressure through the production of specialized hormones that help regulate the size of blood vessel walls as well as salt and water balance in the body. Surrounded by ribs and nestled close to the spinal column, these important organs are well protected from the outside world.

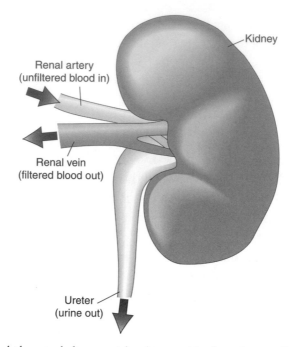

Renal artery
(unfiltered blood in)

Renal vein
(filtered blood out)

Kidney

Ureter
(urine out)

Fig. 1.2. The kidney, including arterial and venous blood supply, as well as the orientation of the renal pelvis and the top of the ureter joining the renal pelvis.

The Renal Pelvis

Like any well-designed factory, the kidney has a production line and factory floor, where the actual product is made. This portion of the kidney is referred to as the *renal parenchyma*, or "meat" of the kidney. The parenchyma is made up of microscopic tubes that filter waste out of the blood and, in the process, create urine. The urine then collects in the central portion of the kidney in a funnel-shaped structure called the *renal pelvis*.

The renal pelvis is different from the rest of the kidney in several important ways. First, it is actually made of different material and performs a completely different function than the meat of the kidney. It is really the starting point of a long pipe system that conveys urine from the production line to the outside world. However, the renal pelvis has nothing to do with the actual production of urine, and loss of all or a portion of it does not usually interfere with the functioning of the associated kidney.

Another differentiating point about the renal pelvis is that the renal pelvis has a thin wall lined with specialized cells that cover the inside of the entire urinary tract all the way to the innermost part of the *urethra*, the tube that carries urine from the bladder during urination. These cells are referred to as *transitional cells* because they actually undergo a transition in appearance, depending upon the amount of fluid in the system and the pressure exerted on the surface of the cells. Cells that line the interior surface of an organ are often called an epithelium. When we talk about transitional cells we often refer to them as the transitional epithelium. It is from these transitional cells that the majority of bladder cancers develop. Cancer in the renal pelvis can also develop from transitional cells, although this occurs infrequently.

The Ureters

The renal pelvis has a special nervous system of its own which contracts at regular intervals to propel urine toward the bladder. From the renal pelvis, urine is carried downstream by the *ureter*, a tubular extension of the renal pelvis with many of the same properties. Each kidney has a renal pelvis that in turn connects to a ureter.

A close anatomic cousin to the renal pelvis, the ureter contracts periodically to propel urine toward the bladder. Unlike the renal pelvis, the ureter is narrow and therefore can easily get kinked or blocked by material that flows with the urine, such as kidney stones or blood clots. The ureters are lined with *transitional epithelium*, a thin layer of tissue. Transitional cell cancers can also develop in this tissue.

The blood supply to the ureter is delicate and has a variety of sources. Injury to the ureteral blood supply can result in scarring and narrowing of the inside diameter of the ureter, which in turn can cause an inhibited flow of urine known as an *obstruction*. Like the renal pelvis, the ureter has nothing to do with actual urine production. However, it is critically important that the ureter function normally: if urine is not transported in a timely fashion, the kidney can become filled with urine, a condition that can compromise normal kidney function and a person's general health.

Obstruction presents two types of problems. First, it can cause the uri-

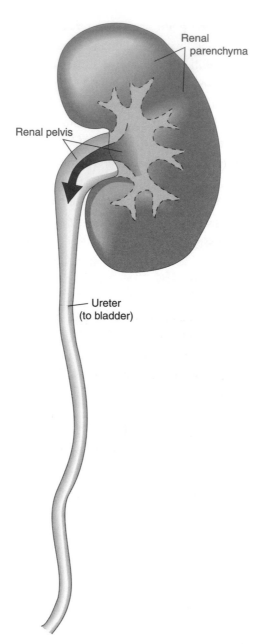

Renal
parenchyma

Renal pelvis

Ureter
(to bladder)

Fig. 1.3. The internal architecture of the kidney and the outflow tract for urine, consisting of the calyces, renal pelvis, and ureter.

nary tract to fill up with an excess amount of fluid. Second, when urine does not flow normally, kidney filtering functions are compromised and the kidney begins to lose its ability to process the waste material in the blood. This is not an immediate event but occurs gradually, over several weeks. If an obstruction is not relieved in an appropriate period of time—usually within a few days and certainly within a week or two—permanent kidney damage results and recovery is almost never complete.

Problems with the kidneys and the urinary tract can generate a great deal of pain. Obstructions cause pain by filling the tubes of the urinary tract with too much fluid. Pressure on the walls of the renal pelvis or the ureter cause a classic form of aching and relentless pain called colic. Patients with kidney stones or some other rapid obstruction of the ureters or other parts of the urinary tract in the upper abdomen can experience a tremendous amount of discomfort that is controlled only with pain medication. Women who have passed kidney stones and also given birth without the benefit of anesthesia will often remark that passing the kidney stone was more painful than having a baby. In contrast to rapid obstruction of the urinary tract, gradual obstruction rarely causes pain. Tumors that slowly obstruct the urinary tract, particularly those of the ureters, can do so without ever causing pain because the obstruction occurs so gradually.

The Bladder

The ureter ends in a connection with the urinary bladder, a muscular, balloonlike structure that sits in the pelvis, the lower part of the trunk of the body. The connection between the ureter and the bladder is called the *ureterovesical junction* (*vesical* means *bladder*). The ureter actually enters the bladder on the bladder's back surface and tunnels into the back of the bladder at its base. This arrangement prevents urine from flowing back toward the kidney when the bladder empties.

The ureterovesical junction and the junction of the ureter and the renal pelvis are the narrowest points between the kidney and the bladder. Typically, these are the places where material can and does get stuck.

The bladder, unlike the thin-walled ureter and renal pelvis, is a thick-walled structure with a heavy muscular coat, and in most people it is sur-

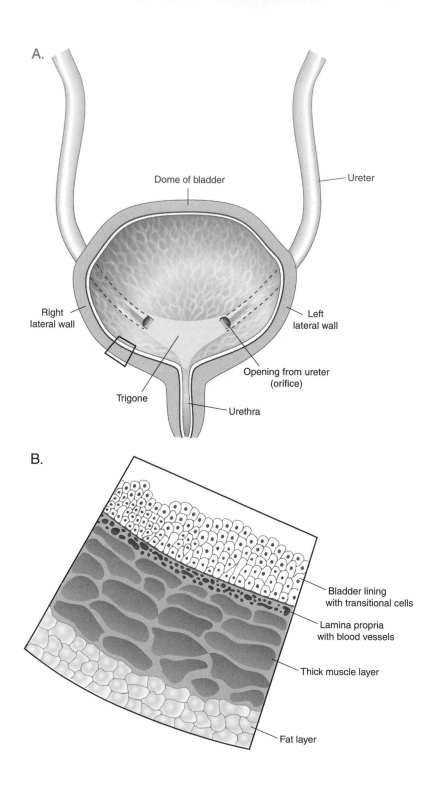

A.

Dome of bladder

Ureter

Right
lateral wall

Left
lateral wall

Opening from ureter
(orifice)

Trigone

Urethra

B.

Bladder lining
with transitional cells

Lamina propria
with blood vessels

Thick muscle layer

Fat layer

rounded by a layer of fat. The muscular covering of the bladder, as you will see, is of tremendous functional and clinical importance. The bladder typically holds 400–500 cubic centimeters (about 1 to 2 pints) of urine. The inner lining of the bladder is composed of transitional cells, and it is thick compared to the wall of the ureter or the wall of the renal pelvis. This means that cancer developing in the lining of the bladder has much farther to go to invade adjacent structures (such as the blood vessels of the pelvis, the rectum, the reproductive organs of women, and the lower portion of the digestive tract) than do tumors arising in either the ureter or the renal pelvis. The *lamina propria* is a specialized layer of blood vessels and cells that separates the lining layer from the actual muscle wall of the bladder.

The bladder expands or contracts according to how much fluid is in it. The muscle of the bladder wall allows the bladder to be forcefully contracted when a person urinates. This contraction, which empties the bladder, is under complex neurologic control that involves the participation of centers in both the brain and the spinal cord. The muscular wall also serves as a barrier through which bladder tumors must grow before they can spread to other regions of the pelvis. While this is not the primary role of the bladder wall, the extent to which the bladder wall is penetrated by bladder cancer is of great importance in deciding what type of therapy is most appropriate. (This will be explained more fully in chapter 3.)

When a urologist examines your bladder with a cystoscope, an instrument that views the interior of the bladder (see chapter 3), there are certain "landmarks" that he or she looks for and uses to describe the location of any abnormalities within the organ. The floor of the bladder is the *trigone*, a triangle-shaped region near the junction of the urethra and the bladder. The walls on either side of the trigone are referred to as the *right* and *left lateral walls*, and the back wall is called the *posterior wall*. The roof of the bladder is called the *dome*.

FACING PAGE:
Fig. 1.4. The internal architecture of the bladder (A), showing a magnified schematic view of the cellular architecture of the bladder wall (B), including the lining with transitional cells, the lamina propria, thick muscle, and covering layer of fat.

The Urethra

The bladder connects to the outside of the body through the urethra, a hollow tube. The structure of the urethra differs somewhat in men and women. In women, the urethra is a relatively short organ that attaches to the bladder neck and is surrounded by muscles that both provide support and constrict the urethra to provide urinary continence, the ability to control the flow of urine. In the male, the urethra is a longer organ and passes through the prostate gland, which surrounds the bladder neck, where the urethra and the bladder are connected. This is an important relationship—the prostate gland and the bladder are intimately connected and really coexist as one organ from a functional standpoint. The prostate plays an important role in male continence, since it is connected to the portion of the bladder neck that provides for involuntary control of urine flow. When a man's prostate has been removed, owing to cancer or for other reasons, he is forced to rely upon the other important component of the urinary control complex, the voluntary sphincter, for urinary continence.

Despite the difference in length, the urethra performs many of the same functions in men and women. The cells that line the urethra change as the urethra travels from the bladder toward the external opening. The cells closest to the bladder are similar to the cells lining the bladder itself, whereas the cells closer to the outside of the body are more like skin. As we will see when we look at cancer in the urinary tract, tumors can arise within the urethra in both men and women, and the location of the tumor frequently determines what cell type the cancer will have, which in turn will direct the type of therapy used to treat a given tumor. In women, the most common urethral cancers are similar to cancers arising on the skin, so-called *squamous cancers*. These tumors are the only kind of urinary tract cancer that occurs more frequently in women than in men. It is particularly important to recognize that *transitional cell cancers* of the urinary tract can occur anywhere along the course of the system, from the renal pelvis and the lining of the kidney to the region where the urethra and the bladder meet, in men or in women.

The Prostate

The prostate is a walnut-sized organ located at the base of the bladder in men. It serves a variety of reproductive and mechanical functions in men. The organ is notable as a common site of cancer in men over the age of 50. In recent years, publicity about the availability of a blood test to check for prostate cancer (the prostate-specific antigen test, PSA) and effective surgical therapies for prostate cancer have made the prostate gland a part of the urinary tract that most people know at least something about.

The prostate gland produces seminal fluid, the liquid that contains the sperm during the process of ejaculation. The prostatic secretions make up the bulk of the fluid of the ejaculate, with the sperm comprising only a small part of the total fluid volume.

Continence and Urinary Control

Continence, as noted above, is the ability to control the flow of urine from the bladder. It is regulated by a complex network of nerves and muscles located in the lower part of the pelvis of both men and women. Despite years of anatomic research into the control and normal function of the bladder and the urethra, the exact mechanisms by which continence is maintained remain incompletely understood. Here is what we do know: In men, urinary control is maintained through the complex interaction of two control mechanisms called *sphincters*. A sphincter is a circular muscle group that effectively cuts off the flow of urine when the muscle is contracting by blocking the urethra or the bladder neck, the region where the bladder and prostate connect. In men, the sphincters are located where the bladder and the prostate join and where the urethra emerges from the substance of the prostate and travels into the penis. The sphincter at the bladder neck is not under voluntary control. When the bladder is filling with urine, reflex nervous impulses travel to and from the bladder and the lower spinal cord.

In addition, messages about bladder volume are transmitted to the brain. This subtle and complex interaction permits fine-tuned regulation of the flow of urine into the urethra. A second sphincter, one that is under voluntary control, is located at the junction of the prostate and the urethra. This second control mechanism is one that a man can voluntarily squeeze when he does not want to urinate. As anyone who has waited too long to go to the bathroom can attest, sometimes the bladder's capacity to empty itself can overcome even the strongest voluntary commands, resulting in incontinence, the leakage of urine.

In women, the control mechanisms are less well defined than they are in men. The female urethra is shorter than the male counterpart, but it performs all of the same functions regarding control of urine flow. It is believed that both voluntary and involuntary control mechanisms exist in women just as they do in men. However, the precise anatomic locations of these structures have been harder to identify. In addition, the nervous system control of the sphincters in women remains controversial and is the subject of ongoing research.

Now that you know a little bit about what a healthy urinary system looks like and where some problems can arise, we will describe a little more about the cancer process and how things can go wrong.

CHAPTER TWO

A Little Background Material

Bladder cancer is a common illness among Americans. A few facts and figures about this disease indicate how prevalent it is and who is most at risk:

—More than 50,000 new cases of bladder cancer will be diagnosed this year.

—About 11,000 people die annually as a direct result of this type of malignancy

—Bladder cancer tends to occur most commonly in people over the age of 60, although it can occur in the very young, including children under 10 years old.

—The disease is about two to three times more common in men than women.

—More Caucasians are affected than African Americans, for reasons that are not known.

These numbers and this type of information compose the *epidemiology* of a disease, the science of who it strikes and how it spreads. Epidemiology is a valuable science that sheds light on what causes diseases and, ultimately, on how to prevent them. As we have already noted, no one knows exactly what causes bladder cancer, but enough epidemiological work has been done so that we are starting to get some ideas about the factors that are involved, at least in some cases.

This chapter is for people who want to know a bit about what doctors and scientists have learned about what causes bladder tumors to develop.

What Causes Bladder Cancer?

Patients frequently ask what causes bladder cancers to develop. Studies to answer this question date from the beginning of the century, when Louis Rehn, a German physician and scientist, established a link between the exposure to chemicals used in the production of colored textiles and the development of bladder cancers in the factory workers who produced these goods. Intense scientific research subsequently revealed that the chemicals, derivatives of a class of compounds called *arylamines*, caused bladder cancers in both experimental animals and in humans exposed to these substances in the workplace.

What has become abundantly apparent through the years is that Rehn's initial observation turns out to be an indictment of sorts of life in the industrialized world of the twentieth century. Many of the wonderful things that make life "better" for those of us who live in industrialized nations—chemicals and the products that are made from or with them—can be linked either directly or, more commonly, indirectly to the development of cancers such as bladder cancer. Although bladder cancers certainly occur in nonindustrialized parts of the world, there seems to be a link in the United States between cancer-causing chemicals and the risk for developing bladder cancer. Ironically, because so many different things could contribute to the development of bladder tumors, it has been difficult for scientists who study disease risk to identify clearly one or another group of substances commonly used by Americans today which is responsible. As is so often the case with this type of complex research, studies both supporting and refuting a given piece of evidence can quickly be found simply by consulting the latest journals.

We can't say, then, that working at a certain job or in a certain environment will definitely result in the development of bladder cancer. We can, however, develop a list of "high-risk" jobs that have been associated with increased bladder cancer risk.

Occupations associated with Risk for Bladder Cancer:

—Dye workers
—Textile workers

—Tire and rubber workers
—Painters
—Truck drivers
—Chemical workers
—Petroleum workers
—Hairdressers
—Aluminum workers

Take this information with a grain of salt, however. During a recent lecture, a slide was projected showing a table of substances thought to increase the risk of bladder cancer. Someone in the audience was kind enough to point out that the list contained tap water. This is a good example, perhaps, of the fact that not all information is useful, even if it appears in a scientific journal or presentation.

Risk Factors

Smokers Beware!

There are things that some people do that probably significantly increase their risk of developing bladder cancer, and there is little argument among scientists and physicians about at least one of these: cigarette smoking is strongly associated with the development of bladder cancer. (Pipe and cigar use are not as clearly related to developing these tumors.) Cigarette smokers have about a two or three times greater risk of developing cancer of the bladder compared to nonsmokers. Though quitting is associated with a decrease in the risk, it can take as long as twenty years to get back to the risk level enjoyed by people who never smoked.

Smokers might find smoking less appealing if they knew that some of the chemicals in cigarette smoke are the same as or related to those that Dr. Rehn and his colleagues found caused cancer in the German textile-industry workers, the aromatic amines. People who have cancer often ask how they can lower their children's risk of developing cancer in the future. Probably the single most important thing you can do is to keep your children or grandchildren from smoking cigarettes. If genetics plays any part in the development of bladder cancer, there's very little you can do now to change your own or your children's genes. But you can impress upon the next generation that not only is smoking not fashionable, it is decidedly dangerous.

What about Changing My Diet?

Many people worry about what they eat and may particularly focus on diet once cancer has been diagnosed. A number of different foods and beverages have been studied to try to learn if they are linked to bladder cancer. Fatty foods and high cholesterol intake, which are bad for your heart, have also been found to contribute to bladder cancer growth. Most studies that have examined coffee and alcohol use have failed to demonstrate a definitive link between these commonly consumed beverages and bladder cancer. Artificial sweeteners have also come in for their share of criticism in this connection, but most well-done research fails to implicate the sugar substitutes in the development of bladder tumors.

People often ask if there are any foods that appear to protect against bladder cancer. The answer is that we are not sure. However, some studies have found that increased consumption of vitamin A and foods that contain carotene appears to lower the rate of bladder cancer. Further research is necessary before we can know for sure what the connection is between these foods and vitamins and the risk of bladder cancer.

Anything Else to Worry About?

Certain medical conditions make people more likely to develop bladder cancer, because of either the condition itself or its treatment. One example is chronic bladder infection with schistosomiasis, a parasite that is common in Egypt and other parts of Africa. Parasitic worms that live in water gain access to the human bloodstream through the skin of the feet and establish themselves in the blood vessels of the pelvis, which supply blood to the bladder. Chronic infection of the bladder tissues over time causes the development of one form of bladder cancer that can be very aggressive. This mechanism of bladder cancer development is virtually unheard of in the United States but is the most common way people get bladder cancer in Egypt.

Some people with paraplegia who have lost normal control of the bladder for neurologic reasons have chronic bladder infection. They must drain their bladder with a catheter, and the irritation caused by the constant catheter use can cause tumors to develop in the lining of the bladder over time. This process usually takes years but can be very serious and requires extensive therapy to correct.

Bladder cancer may also develop as an unfortunate side effect of therapies we use to treat other tumors. High-dose radiation therapy to the pelvis for the primary treatment of cervical cancer has been associated with bladder cancer development. A commonly used and very valuable anticancer drug called *cyclophosphamide* has also been associated with bladder cancer development. To decrease the risk of this drug causing tumors of the bladder, special precautions are now taken during drug administration to ensure that the drug spends little time in contact with the sensitive lining cells of the bladder, where most if not all bladder tumors begin.

Familial Bladder Cancer

Bladder cancer occasionally appears to run in families, although examples of this in the medical literature are rare. Some families have multiple members with bladder cancer, occurring in several generations, while other families have one or two members with bladder cancer and others with other types of cancer. A family tree of one such family appears below. Note that not everyone in this family has bladder cancer, although a number of cases of cancer have been discovered from generation to generation. In this family, a specific type of abnormality of certain genes was discovered. It remains unclear whether this abnormality played any role in the development of cancer in the members of this family. Establishing a specific genetic or environmental cause in families with multiple bladder cancer cases has been generally difficult, and currently families with one member who develops bladder cancer are not thought to be at unusual risk for bladder cancer in subsequent generations.

Genes and DNA

One of the objectives of this book is to get you started on the journey of understanding a complex disease. This can be difficult—remember, this is

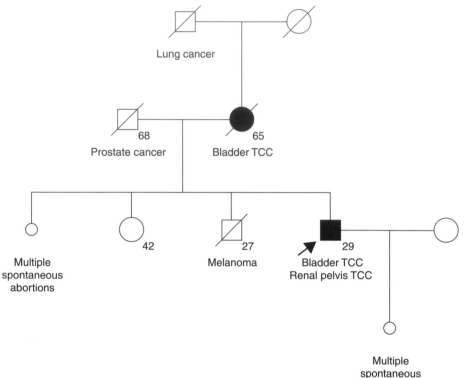

Fig. 2.1. A schematic family tree for a bladder cancer family. Note that the mother died of bladder cancer at age sixty-five, and her twenty-nine-year-old son subsequently developed both bladder cancer and cancer of the renal pelvis.

a disease that is not completely understood even by people who study it for a living. However, current and ongoing research is teaching us about how bladder cancers develop, and this information, in turn, is helping to change the way we treat patients.

To start out, it will be helpful to remember a few things you learned in school and then build on this basic knowledge about biology, chemistry, and genetics. Cancer is really the uncontrolled growth of cells. Cells are the building blocks of tissues: muscles, bones, skin, and other organs such as the bladder. Cells are little bags of chemicals surrounded by a barrier called a membrane. The membrane lets some things in and keeps others out.

Inside the cell, the chemicals that power cellular function are called *proteins*. Proteins take their "marching orders" from a variety of different superior officers, the most senior of which is *deoxyribonucleic acid,* or *DNA,* the material that we refer to as the blueprint of life. DNA is what *genes* are made of; each human cell contains about 100,000 genes. Genes determine different sorts of things about people such as eye color, hair color, and, sometimes, susceptibility to certain diseases.

To store the tremendous amount of information contained in the cell's DNA, the DNA itself is divided into packages called *chromosomes.* Each of us has twenty-three pairs of chromosomes. Chromosomes are stored in the *nucleus* of the cell, a centrally located compartment that is contained within its own membrane, which keeps it more or less separate from the rest of the inside of the cell. A commonplace analogy may be helpful: Think of DNA as the material from which your wardrobe is made. Genes are the different elements of your wardrobe such as the red socks or paisley bow tie. The chromosomes are your closets and drawers, where you keep your clothing, and, if you keep all your clothes in your bedroom, then your bedroom is the nucleus. Your house is the cell and whoever and whatever is running around outside your bedroom is participating in the normal function of your cell's daily life.

All this basic science is relevant to bladder cancer because scientists have discovered that by examining different parts of individual chromosomes they can sometimes find specific genes that, when changed, contribute to the development of cancers. The notion that genes cause diseases now seems commonplace, although this idea is relatively new in scientific terms. Changes in chromosomes were first thought to play a role in the development of cancer at the beginning of the twentieth century. The field of molecular biology—the study of the molecules and, particularly, the behavior of DNA and the genes made up of DNA—soon developed in the 1950s. DNA itself was described less than fifty years ago. The ability to pinpoint genes has evolved considerably in the last decade, so that it is not unusual to read about the discovery of a new gene associated with a specific disease in the morning newspaper.

In a sense, the search for disease genes actually began with bladder cancer. The first *oncogene,* a specific type of cancer-causing gene, was discov-

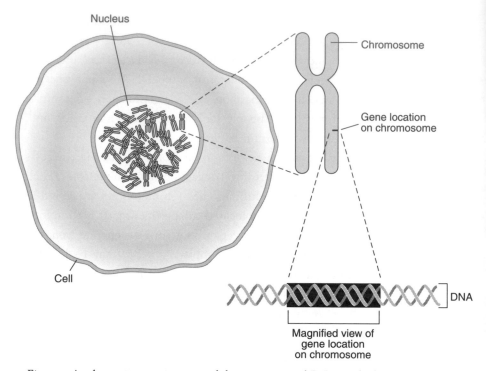

Fig. 2.2. A schematic representation of chromosomes and DNA, with chromosomal location in the cellular nucleus.

ered in a bladder cancer cell. A mutant form of H-*ras*, a gene normally involved in the regulation of cell growth, was discovered in bladder cancer cells kept alive in a dish by means of a technique called tissue culture. *Mutation,* a process in which the normal chemical structure of a gene is altered, leads to a malfunction of the H-*ras* gene, which in turn produces constant stimulation of cell growth. There are a few examples of oncogenes that may play a role in the development of bladder cancer, but we now know that a separate class of genes known as *tumor suppressors* probably play a more central role in the development of cancer.

Tumor suppressor genes are a category of genes thought to be active during development of the embryo and *suppressed* after development is complete. When these genes are lost or inactivated by some means, the molecular "brake" that prevents their growth-stimulating properties is released and cells grow uncontrollably, producing a cancer. By looking around at the different chromosomes using specific laboratory techniques, scientists have been able to identify certain genes (or areas where certain genes ought to be) that appear to be missing or mutated in bladder cancer cells. These techniques identify the location or "home addresses" of specific tumor suppressor genes that play an integral role in tumor development and growth.

The most commonly affected chromosome in bladder cancer is chromosome number 9, and scientists currently believe that disrupting of normal genes on this chromosome leads to the first stages of bladder cancer development. Meanwhile, other chromosomes house other genes that participate in the development of bladder tumors. One of the most important, and one that scientists are learning a great deal about, is the p53 tumor suppressor gene located on chromosome 17.

Every year, the distinguished scientific journal *Science* chooses a "molecule of the year." A few years ago p53 got the honor, but this gene has been in the spotlight for a while. The p53 gene plays a central role in the way normal cells recover after their DNA has been damaged, an event that can happen from such seemingly innocuous insults as sunburn or smoking just one cigarette. Think of someone letting a bushel of hungry moths loose in your clothes closet. Inevitably, no matter how quickly you call the exterminator, some of your wardrobe is going to get damaged, and you're going to have to repair the mess. The p53 gene functions like an in-house exterminator, minimizing the damage done and giving you time to sew up the holes in your new suit. If you lose your p53 gene or for some reason it stops working efficiently, you can sustain a tremendous amount of DNA damage and not have the means to repair it. The damaged DNA gets passed on to other cells in the process of cell division, and a tumor starts to grow. The p53 gene is lost or functions poorly in many advanced bladder cancers. In fact, whether a person's tumor has normal or abnormal p53 function is now being used to determine if the person needs specific types of therapy for cancer.

It is unlikely that the solutions to the mystery of the cause of bladder cancer are as simple as a single gene. Most scientists now believe that bladder cancer is the result of *multiple* genetic—that is, gene-disturbing—

events. Some of this information is being used to develop new tests to detect bladder tumors, while other observations are being evaluated as potential guides for determining which therapies should work best for which patients. We are at the beginning of our search to identify and locate bladder cancer–causing genes, and the results look very promising. However, it will be some time before this type of information can be put to use, and even longer before the *manipulation of defective genes*—so-called gene therapy—can be expected to improve the care of our patients.

Translational Research: Bringing Laboratory Discoveries to the Bedside

Some of the most exciting developments in the area of basic research on bladder cancer involve the application of laboratory techniques to identify bladder cancer cells or substances produced by bladder cancers that are released into the urine. One of the first tests to be developed in the early 1990s is called the BTA (bladder tumor antigen) test. Many other tests have been developed subsequently (FDP, NMP-22, telomerase, and microsatellite assays to name just a few); all detect proteins, enzyme activities, or even DNA structural abnormalities that are characteristic of cancer cells in urine. These novel laboratory tests have two significant potential uses in the context of caring for patients with bladder cancers. For starters, these noninvasive tests (all are performed on voided urine samples) may permit the diagnosis of a tumor without actual insertion of an instrument into the urinary tract. Second, these tests are generally inexpensive, and some can be rapidly performed in a doctor's office. In the future, these tests may be incorporated into standard management protocols for patients at risk for bladder cancer development or recurrence after treatment. Perhaps a sufficiently sensitive and specific test will ultimately be designed that will make routine cystoscopy unnecessary.

If we look at the basic science underlying bladder cancer, we can appreciate that bladder cancer is a complex disease. Evidence suggests that it occurs as a consequence of environmental factors—for example, cancer-causing chemicals—interacting with specific, sensitive genetic locations in our DNA, causing abnormal cell growth. Cessation of smoking can certainly reduce the risk of developing bladder cancer; the importance of modifying diet seems less clear. No one is sure if certain vitamins will prevent bladder cancer, although there are reputable scientists testing this hypothesis. It is important to state that the majority of bladder cancers can be controlled or cured without significant harm to the patient.

In the next chapter, we will introduce you to the signs and symptoms of bladder tumors as well as the tests that are routinely performed to find these cancers and determine the best course of treatment.

CHAPTER THREE

Signs and Symptoms, Tests and Machines

In this chapter, we describe the signs and symptoms of bladder cancer. A sign—more properly, a *clinical sign*—is something physical, such as fever, that patients and doctors can observe. A symptom is something, such as pain, that the patient experiences. Medical evaluation of the these specific signs and symptoms leads to the diagnosis of bladder tumors. Among the techniques used for diagnosis are various types of imaging studies, including conventional x-rays and examinations using specially designed scopes—instruments with lights and optical attachments which are used to evaluate the inside of the bladder. We also describe the methods employed by physicians who analyze bladder tumor biopsies. This is particularly important to understand because most bladder cancer therapy decisions are based on what the microscopic analysis of tumor tissue reveals. Finally, we explain the concept of staging, the clinical science of establishing the location and extent of tumor growth, another significant factor in determining treatment.

Signs and Symptoms

Most people with bladder cancer start out experiencing similar signs and symptoms.

For the majority of people with bladder cancer, the first indication of their condition is *hematuria*, a condition in which blood appears in the urine. Hematuria is classified as either *gross* or *microscopic*; gross means it is visible to the naked eye, without the aid of special equipment, and microscopic means the blood is only visible if a sample of urine is examined using a magnifying device such as a microscope. The presence of blood in the urine is a clinical sign.

While most people with bladder cancer have blood in their urine at some time in the course of their illness, many experience gross hematuria from time to time. Or, the tumor that causes the bleeding may bleed occasionally but not all the time, allowing a person to think, mistakenly, that the problem has gone away. The person with hematuria can also be lulled into a false sense of security because the bleeding associated with most bladder tumors is completely painless. What would you do if you observed blood in your urine one night but experienced no pain and noticed the blood stopped appearing on its own within a short period of time? Not surprisingly, different people react differently. Some feel alarmed and seek immediate medical attention, while others are glad that the bleeding stopped and, not wanting to be "hypochondriacs," go about their business. Yet people who prefer to go about their business usually do come in for testing at the insistence of their spouses or family doctors after several episodes of bleeding have occurred.

> When all this started, my first symptoms were bleeding when I urinated. No pain, just all the sudden, boom!—a lot of blood in my urine. I'd never had anything like this before.
>
> I suddenly noticed during urination that it all came out as blood! That was scary!

Microscopic hematuria is often picked up on routine physical examinations performed by the family doctor. Most annual physical examinations include a urinalysis, in which a specimen of urine is submitted for chemical tests to check for abnormalities such as too much sugar, which could indicate the development of diabetes. One of the routine tests run on urine is a search for red blood cells in the urine, which might signal the presence of disease in the urinary tract. Not all bladder tumors produce enough blood for a person to see, and the search for blood in the urine using special chemical and microscopic analysis occasionally detects tumors that would otherwise go unnoticed until much later in their development. Studies have shown that routine urine testing can catch tumors in early stages, before they become difficult to treat.

Blood in the urine does not automatically mean a diagnosis of cancer, however. Infections, stones, and inflammatory conditions can also cause bleeding. In fact, the vast majority of people with microscopic hematuria are not found to have anything substantially wrong with their urinary tracts. This means that many people are put through numerous tests to find a relatively small number of cancers. The justification for this is that the tests are not overly uncomfortable and the cancers that are found are worth detecting early, in the hope of curing them with minimal risk and inconvenience to the patient.

In addition to the signs, there are also symptoms of bladder cancer you should be aware of. Irritation or pain during urination can indicate the presence of a bladder tumor, although pain is less characteristic of cancer than bleeding. Frequent urination, urgency, and a sensation of always needing to empty the bladder are other symptoms that may be an indication of bladder cancer. Some people with bladder cancer are first thought to have urinary tract infections, and they are frequently treated with antibiotics for some period of time before their symptoms of pain and urgency are recognized as indicators of cancer.

Fever is rarely associated with bladder cancer, and most bladder cancers do not cause rectal bleeding or problems with bowel function. Women who are still menstruating or who have had many urinary tract infections are somewhat less likely to pay attention to pain in the urinary tract or a small amount of visible bleeding. However, these symptoms should not be ignored. Hematuria and urinary tract pain should be discussed with your doctor promptly.

Once a suspicious sign or symptom related to the urinary tract is identified, a person is usually referred to a urologist for evaluation. Although each doctor has his or her own system for evaluating signs and symptoms of urinary tract disease, the evaluation of hematuria is fairly standard and is performed routinely by most urologists. Each patient undergoes a complete medical history and physical examination with particular emphasis placed on the urinary tract. The doctor often asks about medications the patient is taking, because some medications can cause bleeding or other symp-

Table 3.1 Signs and Symptoms of Bladder Cancer

Hematuria (blood in urine)
   Microscopic
   Gross
Irritative urination symptoms
   Pain
   Burning
   Frequency
   Incomplete emptying
Passage of tissue fragments in urine

toms. For example, some blood-thinning medications used by patients with a history of stroke can cause urinary tract bleeding. Other possible medicinal causes include high doses of aspirin used to treat certain types of arthritis.

After taking the medical history, the urologist will examine a urine specimen and check for evidence of blood and signs of infection. Hematuria is also a sign of possible urinary tract infection, so most urologists who evaluate a patient with hematuria will try to rule out a urinary tract infection by performing a urinalysis and a urine culture. The urinalysis will detect the presence of red and white blood cells. White blood cells are specialized infection-fighting cells which enter the urinary tract whenever bacteria attempt to attack the system. The presence of white blood cells in the urine does not rule out bladder cancer, however, since these cells are also present in the urine of some people who have bladder tumors. Therefore a culture—a study of the urine designed to detect bacteria—is also performed. If the culture fails to turn up bacteria or another organism, like yeast, to account for the white blood cells, then additional tests are needed to explain what is going on in the urinary tract. The next step in the evaluation is a specialized form of x-ray called an *intravenous pyelogram*, or *IVP*.

IVP

An intravenous pyelogram is a test that uses dye to examine the kidneys, ureters, and bladder by means of conventional x-rays. People with transitional-cell cancer of the bladder (see chapter 2) may have other

areas of cancer in the transitional cells of the collecting system of the kidneys or in the ureters. The IVP is especially good at finding small cancers
in the upper portions of the urinary tract, especially within the kidney and
ureter. The IVP detects cancers in places that cystoscopy and CT scans
(both explained below) cannot see well. An IVP test usually lasts just under one hour; however, it may take considerably longer if the kidneys function slowly or are not quick to drain.

The first step of the IVP procedure is to inject a dye containing iodine
through a small vein in the hand or arm. This dye mixes with the blood
and circulates through the body to the kidneys. The kidneys, as part of
their cleansing and filtering function, extract the dye from the blood.
Within minutes of the dye injection, several x-ray pictures are taken. In
them, the concentrated dye "lights up" the kidneys. The dye passes from
the kidneys into the urine and follows the usual route that urine takes.
The dye then illuminates the collecting system of the kidneys, the ureters,
and the bladder. The radiologist, a doctor whose specialty is understanding
and interpreting imaging tests, evaluates the pictures for abnormal areas
of blockage or growths.

The evening before an IVP examination, you should eat a light dinner.
To prepare for an IVP, your doctor may ask you to cleanse your bowels the
evening before the study by drinking fluids containing citrate of magne-
sium. Emptying your bowels as much as possible is essential because full
bowels may obstruct your doctor's view of the kidneys. The morning of the
exam, take all your usual medications with some sips of water. You will be
instructed to skip breakfast. Call ahead and check with your doctor or the
radiology team if you take certain medications that must be taken with
food. If you have diabetes, ask your doctor if any adjustments need to be
made in your medications. One oral diabetes medication, called gluco-
phage or metformin, is often stopped several days before the IVP. Ask your
doctor before stopping or altering any of your medicines.

When you arrive at the radiology suite, you will fill out a questionnaire
or form. The radiologist who is responsible for your care that day may be
unfamiliar with your background, and this form protects you by letting
him or her know more about your medical history. Certain medical conditions may require alterations in the way your urinary tract is evaluated.
Some of those medical conditions are listed below:

1. Allergy to dye: If you have received the IVP dye before and were told you had an allergic reaction to the dye, you must tell this to the radiologist. If you have had an allergic reaction, you may not be eligible for the IVP, or there may be special medicines you have to take before the IVP. Allergic reactions to the IVP dye include hives, itching, sneezing, wheezing, or anaphylaxis. These allergic reactions occur within minutes after receiving the IVP dye.

2. Diabetes mellitus, taking pills to control blood sugar: If you have this condition, your renal function may be decreased. The radiologist may adjust the amount of the IVP dye you receive, or you may not be eligible for the IVP.

3. Pregnancy: Usually, patients who are pregnant should not receive the IVP unless it cannot be postponed until after pregnancy.

4. Asthma: Persons who have asthma or other allergic conditions are slightly more likely to have an allergy to IVP dye than those persons who do not have asthma.

5. Multiple myeloma: Patients who have this condition of the bone marrow should not receive IVP dye.

6. Sickle cell disease: Patients with sickle cell disease often have decreased renal function; the dose of the IVP dye may have to be adjusted.

7. Pheochromocytoma or adrenal tumor: These conditions may raise blood pressure during the IVP study.

8. Kidney disease or kidney failure: Patients with these conditions will receive a lower dose of IVP dye. With renal failure, the kidneys do not remove the IVP dye from the body very quickly.

If you have a history of allergic reactions to dye, discuss this with either your primary care doctor or the radiologist a few days before the appointment for the IVP. People with this history are often asked to take steroid pills (for example, prednisone) as a preventive measure to protect against allergic reaction. If you have a history of anaphylaxis (see below), this also should be discussed with your primary doctor and the radiologist.

After reading your answers on the questionnaire, the radiologist will speak with you about your medical history. He or she will then discuss the importance of the test and its possible side effects and risks. Risks include the possibility of some "allergic" reactions to the dye like sneezing, itching, or hives. In the rarest of cases, people have become seriously ill from intravenous dye. This serious illness, called *anaphylaxis*, causes the mouth and windpipe to swell and may cause blockage. The risk of anaphylactic reaction (about 1 in 40,000 to 100,000 persons) or death is comparable to the chance of a fatal auto accident in city driving. Trained personnel are on hand whenever dye is given, to provide treatment if a patient were to have an adverse reaction.

Make sure to ask any questions you have about the procedure. (Many patients find that it's a good idea to jot down questions in a notepad in the days before a medical test or examination.) After all of your questions have been answered, you will be asked to change out of your clothes and put on a patient gown. This protects your clothing from being soiled and prevents any buttons or zippers from appearing on the final x-ray pictures. Be aware that the IVP rooms are often cold, unfortunately, in part because the machines function better with cooler temperatures.

The entire IVP test takes place while you are lying on a table. If you are uncomfortable for any reason, let the technologist know so he or she can make you more comfortable. A nurse or doctor slides the tip of a small catheter, or needle, into a vein in your hand or arm. The doctor or nurse then injects about three ounces of liquid dye into the catheter in your vein.

> The IVP test didn't hurt at all. None of the diagnostic tests hurt, there really wasn't even much discomfort. I was fine.

Once the injection begins, most people feel flushed, a warm sensation throughout their bodies. People also experience a metallic taste in their mouths. Both of these feelings are normal and last for only a few minutes. Some people experience a warm feeling in their arm, but the injection of dye should not be painful. Years ago, many people experienced nausea when given dye, but the dyes have been improved and this now happens much less often. Let the physician or technologist know if you have any unusual feelings at all, especially if you experience itchiness, difficulty in breathing, or nausea.

Suspended from the ceiling above you is a large machine that contains

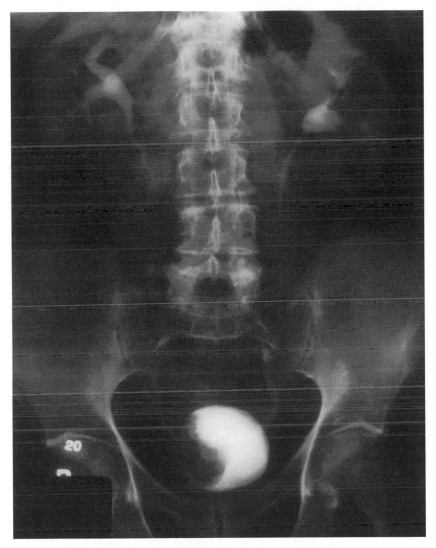

Fig. 3.1. An intravenous urogram, also known as an IVP. Note that the large, dark defect on the left side of the bladder image, corresponding to the right side of the patient's bladder, is in fact a large tumor filling approximately one-third of the volume of the patient's bladder. The kidneys and ureters in this patient are normal. The bony structures of the back and pelvis are also clearly noted on the x-ray.

the x-ray tube. It spins during the procedure and may make a loud whirring noise. It may seem a bit dangerous, but there is little risk—the machine is tightly fastened to the ceiling and it is supposed to move a little. The loud noise and unexpected motion may be startling.

As part of the procedure, a wide belt may be put around your waist. It is intended to constrict the area underneath your kidneys, in order to hold the urine. The belt needs to be tight to hold the urine up in your kidneys, but it should not hurt. The belt can be adjusted if it is too tight.

Toward the end of the IVP test, you will be asked to get up and empty your bladder by urinating. One final x-ray picture will be taken, and then you will be finished and free to resume all normal activities.

Cystoscopy

Though x-rays can tell us something about the lining of the bladder, the "gold standard" for the evaluation of the lower urinary tract is direct visual examination with a specialized instrument called a *cystoscope*. The word *cystoscope* comes from the Greek word *cyst*, which means bladder—cystoscopy is examination of the bladder interior with a scope. The purpose of routine outpatient cystoscopy is to evaluate the lining of the lower urinary tract.

Evaluation of the lower urinary tract using scopes is not a new procedure. Physicians in Europe designed various types of "scopes" for inspection of the bladder in the seventeenth century. Those scopes were primarily useful for examining women, because the female urethra is short and the instruments of the day, run on candlepower, could not supply enough light to illuminate the longer male urethra. Later, in the early part of the twentieth century, scopes used to inspect the bladder were aided by small electric lightbulbs. The view of the bladder was better than that provided by candlelight, but the bulbs were fragile and had an annoying habit of burning out in the middle of examinations. The cystoscope used today was invented in the 1960s. With light provided by reliable, high-power energy sources, state-of-the-art fiberoptic equipment that can provide an excellent view of the entire bladder interior is available in virtually every urologist's office.

There is little or no preparation necessary for the patient undergoing routine outpatient diagnostic cystoscopy. This is a relatively simple procedure that is performed in an examining room with only local anesthetic. However, there are a few things that will be helpful to keep in mind once you have learned you will need cystoscopy. No one likes to have things "done" to his or her body. Nonetheless, anticipation is frequently the worst part of any medical procedure. Most men and many women approach the prospect of having a small scope introduced into the urethra with trepidation. The best way to lessen your fears is to know exactly what to expect. Our patients usually tell us after the procedure that they only experienced minimal discomfort and it was not as bad as they had expected.

The cystoscope is introduced into the urethra as the patient lies on his or her back. Different models of cystoscopy equipment may require slightly different positioning of the legs during the examination. With the scope that we use most often, men lie flat on their backs and women rest their legs in a set of stirrups similar to those used by gynecologists for performing pelvic examinations.

We prepare our patients for cystoscopy by first asking them to remove their clothes and put on a gown. Then the patient is asked to lie on an examination table, as described above, either flat on his back or with her legs resting in stirrups. The genitalia are washed with antibiotic soap to minimize the risk of an infection at the time of the procedure. Sterile drapes or sheets are placed over the patient's body to keep the area clean during the examination. A jellylike substance (similar in consistency to K-Y lubricant) containing lidocaine, a numbing medicine, is squirted into the urethra. The lubricant makes the urethra slippery, easing the passage of the scope into the bladder. The anesthetic removes some of the discomfort associated with the passage of the scope and makes the examination more tolerable for most patients.

Many patients ask, in worried anticipation of cystoscopy, if the examination can be done under general anesthesia. In the past, diagnostic cystoscopy on adults was sometimes performed under general anesthesia; today, however, general anesthesia is rarely used for this examination, and only if there are unusual medical circumstances. Fear and anxiety are not considered valid reasons for using general anesthesia for cystoscopy. Most insurance companies will not pay for the expense associated with the anes-thesia, and most urologists will tell you that the risk of anesthesia far out-weighs any benefit for what is truly a minor procedure. Some urologists will provide calming medications (for example, Valium) for anxious pa-tients before cystoscopy.

After the lower urinary tract is lubricated and numbed, the cystoscope is inserted into the urethra and carefully advanced into the bladder as the urologist looks through the lens at the end of the instrument. Throughout the examination, the doctor will tell you what he or she is seeing and explain different sensations you may feel during cystoscopy. In most cases, the cystoscope is actually inside a person only three to four minutes.

Cystoscopes come in two varieties. Rigid cystoscopes are the original instruments, which have been used over the past one hundred years to examine the lower urinary tract. These rigid steel instruments are actually very easy to use and are well tolerated by most patients. Some male pa-tients find examinations with this standard type of cystoscope uncomfort-able, and a recent advance has made cystoscopy more comfortable for all patients. The flexible cystoscope is an instrument that can be bent by the urologist to conform to the contours of the body, such as the curving path of the urethra. This is particularly useful in the male patient. The scope's flexibility is made possible by a special lens or optical system called *fiber-optics*, which transmits light through very fine glass fibers from a powerful light source to the inside of the bladder. The result is an instrument that bends with the patient's tissue, in contrast to the old-style rigid scopes, which used to make the patient's tissue bend with the scope. Flexible scopes are widely used by urologists in all settings throughout the United States and represent the most advanced technology in outpatient exami-nation, both for comfort and for the information provided by the instru-ment (see figure 4.1).

One of the major diagnostic advantages of the flexible scope is that it can be "flexed" backward to provide a view of the connection between the bladder and the urethra, the region called the bladder neck. Since the rigid scope cannot be flexed but instead relies for its ability to inspect the blad-der with a series of complex compound lenses that cannot provide a complete view of the bladder neck, tumors and other lesions located at or near the bladder neck are much better seen with the flexible scope.

Patient comfort is an equally compelling reason to use a flexible scope. Flexible examinations usually take less time because the entire examination can be performed with the same lens system, while examinations with a rigid scope require changing the lens system during the study. Both male and female patients prefer the flexible scope because of its narrow diameter and the lower level of discomfort produced by this instrument. Cystoscopy does not have to be a painful or traumatic experience.

Since the urinary tract is both hollow and pliant, the walls of the bladder collapse when this organ is not full of fluid. To get an adequate look at the interior surface of the bladder, the urologist must inflate it. This is usually done with sterile water that is run into the bladder during cystoscopy through the cystoscope itself. You may feel your bladder getting full during the examination. If the pressure becomes uncomfortable, tell your doctor and he or she can let a bit of fluid out of the bladder during the study to make the experience more tolerable.

> The old kind of cystoscope is stiff and rigid. You're more tense than anything else. It's not painful but it's uncomfortable and they try to get it over with as quickly as possible. The newer scope is more flexible. I didn't even know the doctor had started looking. I asked him when he was going to start, and he said he had finished.

During cystoscopy, patients experience a sense of burning or stinging. In general, women seem to tolerate cystoscopy somewhat better than men, probably because they have experienced gynecological exams and are more accustomed to genital examination than men are. In addition, the longer male urethra and the location of the prostate gland at the base of the bladder, where the urethra and the bladder meet, can slightly increase the discomfort of cystoscopy for male patients. Men are sensitive in the area of the prostatic urethra, and many complain of an acute need to urinate during this portion of the procedure. Men also often experience a fleeting sense of burning or irritation in the urethra as the scope passes through the region of the prostate and into the bladder itself. Once the scope is in the bladder, the discomfort diminishes and may disappear completely. Cystoscopy is very well tolerated by most male patients, however, particularly those who know what to expect.

During the exam, the bladder is completely inspected and any abnormalities are noted. Viewing the bladder through a cystoscope is like looking into a fluid-filled balloon. The walls are curved, and any air introduced during the insertion of the cystoscope rises to the top of the inside of the bladder, a region called the dome. Urologists refer to specific bladder features in describing the results of cystoscopy so that other doctors will know the location of any problems discovered during the procedure. The trigone, as explained in chapter 1, is the floor of the bladder, a triangle-shaped region near the junction of the urethra and the bladder. This part of the bladder is where the ureters empty urine from each kidney. Not surprisingly, many bladder tumors arise on or near the trigone, presumably because potentially cancer-causing substances concentrated in the urine are dumped in relatively high concentration onto the tissue of the trigone. The walls on either side of the trigone are referred to as the lateral walls, either right or left, and the back wall is called the posterior wall.

After the exam the doctor will remove the scope, and you will get dressed and meet with the urologist to discuss the results of the study. If no abnormalities are discovered, you can expect a cystoscopy to take about three to five minutes to complete. If abnormalities such as tumors, stones, or patches of apparently abnormal tissue are discovered during cystoscopy, the procedure will take a little longer. A small piece of the abnormal tissue can be removed using special instruments that are passed through the sheath of the cystoscope. This procedure is called a *biopsy*. The material is sent to the pathology laboratory for analysis, and the results of this analysis will help your doctor decide whether to recommend further procedures. Biopsy is a minor surgical procedure that will be explained in greater detail in the following chapter.

Let's look now at findings of diagnostic cystoscopy that might indicate the presence of a bladder tumor. Some bladder tumors look like little bushes, others look like seaweed or small coral formations. Still others look like heaped-up mounds of abnormal bladder tissue, some of which has recently been bleeding. The significance of the different shapes will be explained later in this chapter, in the section on types of bladder cancer. Tumors vary in color from pale pink to yellow to tan. Some are dark purple, particularly if the tumor has recently hemorrhaged (bled). Although the examining urologist can usually assume some things about a tumor just by looking at it, it is extremely difficult to tell much about the tumor without a biopsy.

Sometimes urine from the bladder also is sent for analysis in the cytopathology laboratory, where specialized tests are used to search for evidence of tumor cells that have fallen off and are floating free in the urine itself. This type of analysis is particularly helpful in cases in which the cystoscopic exam is normal and the urologist cannot find a particular physical abnormality to explain a patient's signs or symptoms.

To better understand how specialized tests on tissue and urine samples can aid in the evaluation of patients suspected of having bladder tumors, it is helpful to learn a little about the field of pathology, the study of abnormal or diseased tissues and cells.

From Cystoscopy to Pathology: What the Pathologist Does

Many of us are familiar with pathologists from television shows such as *Quincy* and *Homicide*, which depict pathologists performing postmortem examinations (autopsies) on people whose death was either clearly homicide, suspicious of criminal involvement, or unexpected and sudden. These pathologists are generally medical examiners who have specialized in forensics, one branch of pathology. Although the role of the forensic pathologist is important, pathologists wear many other hats.

Pathologists are physicians who train in this specialty for an additional three to six years after medical school. During their training they cover every organ system and, by meticulously analyzing tissue, learn how to diagnose the many thousands of diseases that affect people. Pathology is divided into two major branches, *clinical pathology* and *anatomic pathology*. Clinical pathologists conduct and report on the numerous laboratory tests that are performed on patients, such as doing a urine culture to detect microorganisms and determining whether there are minute quantities of blood in the urine. The anatomic pathologist practices surgical pathology and cytopathology and performs autopsies in medical cases as well. The practice of medicine by the surgical pathologist and cytopathologist is generally performed behind the scenes. When a doctor finds a mass that looks suspiciously like cancer—whether it be in the breast, colon, bladder, or any other organ—he or she takes a biopsy of the suspicious lesion. All surgical specimens go to the surgical pathology department, where the pathologist analyzes the tissue that has been biopsied. The job of the surgical pathologist is to determine the type of tumor, how extensive it is, whether it has spread to lymph nodes, and, if tumor-removal surgery was done, whether the tumor was totally removed.

Occasionally a patient with a significant sign or symptom of urological disease is found to have a "normal" exam by cystoscope. When this happens, a sample of urine is sent to the lab to ensure that microscopic evidence of cancer cells in the urine is not missed. Since the entire urinary tract is bathed in urine, some of the surface cells are sloughed off into the urine and can be detected in the urine specimen. Examination of the urine specimen is a safe and easy procedure. It is done by a *cytopathologist,* a specialist who has additional training in evaluating specimens from bodily fluids, such as urine and sputum, and in examining cells that have been shed, or "exfoliated," from different parts of the body. A urine examination can be used for initial diagnosis of bladder cancer and also for follow-up, to monitor for recurrence of disease after treatment. The examination of urine by the cytopathologist has not been as effective at detecting early cancer as the Pap smear, a widely used screening test for cancer of the uterine cervix. However, urine cytology is still a valuable adjunct to cystoscopy in the search for bladder cancer.

The Role of Pathologists in Medical and Surgical Cases

The field of surgical pathology evolved out of the growing need for accurate microscopic diagnosis. In the early days of surgery, only the surgeon who performed a procedure would examine the organ that had been removed. Over time, more and more diseases were characterized microscopically, and the complexity of microscopic diagnosis increased. For instance, many varieties of cancer were found, and disease processes other than cancer were found to mimic cancer. It became difficult for surgeons to be competent at surgery, patient care, *and* the increasingly complicated demands of microscopic diagnosis. So now, the pathologist is often the medical expert who is called to make the definitive diagnosis on a case. If you have symptoms of bladder cancer, for example, the urologist may examine you with the cystoscope. If he or she sees a lesion on your bladder, the lesion is biopsied or removed completely, if possible, and sent to the pathology laboratory. Although the surgeon may suspect cancer, there is no way to be sure of the diagnosis until the specimen has been examined microscopically by the pathologist.

The consequences of making an incorrect diagnosis on a patient's biopsy are serious, since the diagnosis often dictates whether a major surgical procedure will be performed. The current standard of care in most places is that, prior to surgery, a surgical pathologist must examine all biopsy specimens. The pathologist is central to patient care, and the surgeon will not act without consulting the pathologist.

When biopsy tissue is obtained, it is first placed in a preservative, which prevents the tissue from undergoing the natural process of decomposition. The preservative maintains the specimen in an intact state so it can be viewed under the microscope. The tissue is then embedded in a solid wax mold. A technician cuts a very thin slice of the wax-embedded tissue and places the tissue on a microscope slide. When the wax is melted away, the tissue sticks to the slide. The tissue, which in its natural state is entirely transparent, is stained with purple and blue dyes and then examined under the microscope by the pathologist. The stained characteristics of the cells in the tissue can be instrumental to establishing a diagnosis.

Occasionally it is necessary to analyze tissue immediately. The "quick and dirty" method of immediate tissue evaluation is called *frozen-section analysis*. Frozen sections are performed during the actual surgery. Often, when a surgeon removes an organ, it cannot be determined whether the cancer that is present in that organ has been entirely removed, and the surgeon calls on the pathologist during surgery to analyze a frozen section. A quick-freezing procedure—usually immersion of the tissue in liquid nitrogen—allows the pathologist to slice the tissue thin enough to rapidly make a useful slide. The pathologist takes a portion of the specimen at the margin of excision and examines it microscopically. If the result shows no cancer, the surgeon can conclude the surgical procedure. If the margin was not free of cancer, the surgeon will attempt to remove additional tissue until only normal tissue remains at the margin.

Determining If Your Biopsy Contains Cancer Cells

Cancer cells appear different from normal cells when viewed under the microscope. The size and shape of cells and the characteristics of the cell nucleus are useful in distinguishing cancer. Imagine a row of aluminum soda cans that are precisely aligned. These are the normal cells. Now imagine partially crushing those cans and then attempting to align them in a row. Imagine also that the shapes of the individual crushed cans are different from each other. This is cancer. This variation in shape is called *pleomorphism*, which means occurring in more than one form. Pleomorphism is a very important diagnostic feature of cancer. The most reliable microscopic change in a cancer cell is a change in the structure of its nucleus, the center of the cell where the genetic material (DNA) is contained. Since cancer is a disease resulting from aberrations in the genetic material of a cell, it is not surprising that the repository for the genetic material, the nucleus, is altered in cancer. In most cases, compared to those of normal cells cancer cell nuclei appear "angry" and pleomorphic, displaying changes in size and shape and staining characteristics of the nuclei. The pathologist is able to analyze the changes in size and shape of the cells using the microscope and different staining techniques. Similar criteria of cellular and nuclear shape and pleomorphism are used to diagnose individual cells or clumps of cells that appear in the urine.

Grade and Stage

Approximately 95 percent of bladder tumors arise from the transitional epithelium. There are two types of cancers that arise from this surface lining: *superficial* and *invasive*. In appearance, each of these can be either *papillary*, a collection of small protruding cells resembling a small bush or shrub, or *flat and low*, like a mound of earth or sand.

Grading and staging are two evaluative measures used to rate tumors. Although it is early in your reading about bladder cancer diagnosis, it is not too early to get a handle on the terms *grade* and *stage*, because they are commonly used and frequently misunderstood. These terms are used to describe different characteristics of bladder tumors:

—*Grade*, expressed as a numeral, refers to the appearance of the tumor under the microscope and increases (from 1 up to 3) as tumor cells lose characteristics of the normal cells from which they evolved.

—*Stage*, also expressed as a numeral, refers to the location of the tumor cells in relation to the lining cells, the muscle wall, and the fat that surrounds the bladder; that is, it expresses how far the cancer cells have spread from the original site.

Stage is the tumor characteristic that often determines what type of therapy a patient will receive. The stage of a bladder cancer is a doctor's best estimate of how extensive the tumor is: how much the tumor has grown and how far it has traveled either within or out of the organ from which it originated. We say *estimate* because clinical staging—the art of assembling all of the studies, biopsies, physical examination findings, and all other available information about a patient and his or her tumor—is an indirect measure of the physical extent of the tumor itself. Pathological staging, the actual physical assessment of a tumor after it has been removed, obviously is only possible during or after surgery. Since the doctor's object is to evaluate every tumor as completely as possible *before* treating the patient, and since the extent of disease has a lot to do with what therapy the doctor recommends for a given patient, clinical staging, that business of educated guessing, is a critical if imprecise part of caring for people with bladder cancers.

One of the original staging systems for bladder tumors was developed more than fifty years ago by Hugh Jewett, a Johns Hopkins urologist. Dr. Jewett and his colleagues recognized that patient survival in cases of bladder cancer depended largely on the extent of disease.

Think of stage as a way of diagraming the three-dimensional location of a tumor in a bladder. The international staging system that most doctors use to describe bladder cancers appears in Table 3.2. Basically, stage Ta is

Table 3.2 International Staging System for Bladder Cancer

T-Tumor:

TX	Primary tumor cannot be evaluated
T0	No primary tumor
Ta	Noninvasive papillary carcinoma
TIS	Carcinoma in situ ("flat tumor")
T_1	Tumor invades connective tissue under the epithelium (surface layer)
T_2	Tumor invades muscle
	T_2a Superficial muscle affected (inner half)
	T_2b Deep muscle affected (outer half)
T_3	Tumor invades perivesical (around the bladder) fatty tissue
	T_3a microscopically
	T_3b macroscopically (e.g., visible tumor mass on the outer bladder tissue)
T_4	Tumor invades any of the following: prostate, uterus, vagina, pelvic wall, abdominal wall

very early cancer that has not grown away from its original site on the inner lining of the bladder. This is called *superficial cancer*. Another form of superficial cancer is *carcinoma in situ* (stage TIS), which is an aggressive form of superficial disease with all of the adverse cellular characteristics of invasive cancers. However, although it can spread rapidly and unpredictably, carcinoma in situ, or CIS, as it is known, has not invaded the *lamina propria*, the specialized layer of blood vessels and cells that separates the lining layer from the actual muscle wall of the bladder. Stage T_1 means that cancer cells have spread deeper into the bladder's inner lining but not into the muscular wall of the bladder. In stage T_2 bladder cancers, the cancer has spread to the muscle of the wall of the bladder, and in stage T_3 the cancer cells have moved throughout the bladder wall and spread to the outer tissues that surround the bladder or into the abdomen and nearby reproductive organs. In stage T_4, cancer cells are found on the wall of the abdomen or pelvis or in lymph nodes in the area, sometimes invading other parts of the body.

The majority of bladder cancers arise from the lining cells of the bladder. Over 75 percent of these tumors remain confined to the lining layer and do not invade the bladder wall. These noninvasive tumors are called *superficial transitional cell cancers* and are associated with an extremely favorable overall prognosis. Superficial tumors are usually of a low grade, and although they have a significant tendency to recur, these cancers fortunately do not frequently progress to more aggressive lesions. In fact, only about 10 percent of superficial bladder cancers get worse and require extensive therapy during the life of the patient. Most superficial lesions can be treated and controlled using a special type of cystoscope equipped with an electrical knife used to remove these tumors. Most tumors that are successfully removed with a scope are classified as Ta cancers in the international classification. In addition to using the scope, different drugs can be placed inside the bladder to control the recurrence of superficial bladder tumors. Chapter 4 details scope surgery and medical therapy for superficial tumors.

In contrast to superficial tumors, bladder cancers that grow into the wall of the bladder are considered invasive and require more aggressive therapy. Tumors that leave the lining of the bladder must first penetrate the lamina propria. To visualize this, picture a horizontal brick wall resting on a slab of concrete that in turn is resting on the ground. The bricks in the wall are the lining cells of the bladder, the cement slab separating the cells from the ground is the lamina propria, and the ground is the muscle of the bladder wall. The lamina propria is an important layer because it represents the last barrier many tumors cross as they develop the capacity to get out of the bladder and spread to other parts of the body. Lamina propria tumors are called *superficially invasive* because, although these tumors do not actually reach the true muscle of the bladder wall, they frequently have aggressive cellular characteristics (that is, they are often grade 3) and do not always respond to the types of conservative therapy used routinely for Ta tumors.

Once a tumor has penetrated the lamina propria, it proceeds into the muscle layer of the bladder. This layer is thick in comparison to the lining layer or the lamina propria, a fact that works in the patient's favor. Tumors that invade the bladder wall musculature are called T_2 tumors. If only the innermost layer of the muscle has been penetrated by the tumor, then the tumor is referred to as T_2a, whereas tumors that show deep muscle penetration are called T_2b. As long as the tumor has not traveled completely through the bladder wall to the fat layer on the outer surface of the organ, the tumor remains T_2. Once the tumor extends to the bladder's fat covering, it is designated T_3. As mentioned above, if adjacent organs such as the prostate, vagina, or rectum are affected by the tumors, the stage is T_4.

Before leaving the discussion of staging for the moment, one last detail should be addressed. *Lymph nodes* are storehouses for white blood cells, which fight infection and other types of disease. These critical structures serve as outposts of defense throughout the body and are often the first site to which a tumor spreads when cancer leaves its organ of origin and sets up housekeeping elsewhere. There are many lymph nodes in the pelvis near the bladder. These are some of the first sites bladder cancers will migrate to. Lymph nodes are routinely sampled during bladder cancer surgery to determine whether or not microscopic evidence of tumor spread is present; such evidence could potentially change the management of an individual patient's care.

Radiological Evaluations

Having covered this background information about the importance of staging, let's move on to look at the additional tests used to establish, as best we can, an individual patient's disease stage. Rather than opening up the human body with a knife, specialized radiological studies are the best methods to determine stage; these studies can produce images of the internal organs and frequently provide important information about the extent of tumor growth. The studies we use most commonly are *ultrasonography* (US), *computed tomography scanning* (CT scan) and *magnetic resonance imaging* (MRI). When patients have symptoms that suggest that some part of their bony skeleton may have bladder tumor cells in it, another helpful study is *bone scanning*.

Ultrasonography

Ultrasonography, or ultrasound imaging, creates pictures of the urinary tract in a safe and painless way. Ultrasound is a noninvasive, patient-friendly test with no known side effects or adverse reactions. No bladder catheters or intravenous catheters or any other invasive tools are needed.

Throughout the test the patient simply reclines on a bed in a quiet, dark room. An ultrasound study of the kidneys and bladder usually takes about 30 minutes.

To begin the ultrasound procedure, the technologist applies a warm gel to the patient's abdomen or side and then places a hand-held probe on the patient's skin. The technologist points this probe toward an internal organ like the bladder. The probe has several functions. It sends out sound waves that travel through the patient's body and bounce off internal organs, creating echoes. These sound echoes are like the echoes you might hear when shouting at the edge of a canyon, but they are at a frequency that humans cannot hear. The probe also acts as a receiver, which "hears" the echoes. The echoes are translated to form pictures of the bladder and kidneys on a video screen.

Ultrasound imaging can locate very slight blockages of the urinary tract and blood clots or stones in the bladder. It also measures the thickness of the bladder wall. Ultrasound waves travel best through fluid, so about an hour before the study you will be asked to drink fluids to fill your bladder. Beginning about an hour before your ultrasound appointment, you should also try to hold off going to the bathroom in order to keep your bladder full. If your bladder is nearly full when you arrive, you will have a shorter waiting time before the ultrasound begins.

The positive aspects of ultrasound are its noninvasiveness and its lack of radiation. However, it is limited in that it cannot provide the fine detail that surgeons require before performing an operation. Because small tumors within the collecting system, within the kidneys, and within the ureters may not be seen, other imaging studies may also be needed.

CT Scanning

CT scanning, an abbreviation for computed tomographic scanning (sometimes called "CAT" scanning, for *computed axial tomographic scanning*) creates very detailed pictures of the body using a sophisticated system of x-ray images. The CT pictures show detailed anatomy of the internal organs like the liver and lungs, bones, blood vessels, and soft tissues like lymph nodes. Because it shows these parts of the body well, CT scanning helps doctors see if a cancer has spread. In patients with bladder cancer,

CT scans are used for staging, to thoroughly search for cancer outside of the bladder, and to help determine the most appropriate therapy.

A team consisting of radiologists (doctors who specialize in imaging the body), technologists, and nurses work together to care for you during this study. Plan on being in the CT area for about one hour. The scan itself lasts about ten to fifteen minutes. In preparation for your CT scan, most radiologists recommend not eating or drinking for eight hours prior to the test. This is because food in your stomach gets in the way of the CT pictures.

Empty your bladder after you check in and register so you will be comfortable during the exam. When you arrive at the radiology suite, you will

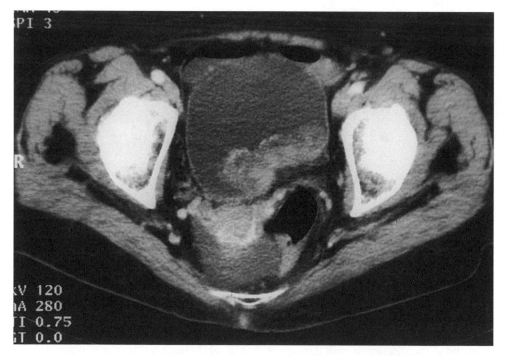

Fig. 3.2. A CT scan of the pelvis indicates a large bladder tumor invading the base of this patient's bladder. The bladder is visible at the bottom center of the scan. The tumor tissue appears as cloudy material within the bladder, while remaining space in the bladder is eclipsed—seen here as the dark area just right of center. The tumor appears to be muscle-invasive based on this CT scan.

fill out a questionnaire or form to provide the radiologist with your medical history. Certain medical conditions may require alterations in the way your urinary tract is evaluated. These are the same medical conditions that were discussed above in the section about the IVP. After reading the form, the radiologist will ask you about your medical history. He or she will then discuss the test and its possible side effects and risks.

Before the test, you will be asked to drink several glasses of a chalky liquid. This liquid is an oral dye that contains either iodine or barium. The dye fills your stomach and intestines so it will be easier to distinguish normal organs from abnormal. It is necessary to finish all of the liquid so your intestines will be full all the way down into the pelvis. You may be asked to wear a patient gown, because metal objects on your clothing or accessories can cast shadows on the CT pictures.

During the scan you will be alone in the room. Most rooms have audio systems and large windows or closed-circuit TV cameras. The technologist will speak to you through a microphone and watch and listen to you throughout the scan.

You will lie on your back on a table for the CT scan. While lying on the table, you will be moved through the CT tube. The doctor or nurse will inject another dye, three ounces of an iodine-based dye, into your hand or arm vein. After the dye is injected, the study takes approximately five minutes. Once the injection begins, most people feel warm sensations through their body and experience a metallic taste in their mouths. Both of these are normal, and the injection of dye should not be painful. Let the physician or technologist know if you have any unusual feelings at all, especially itchiness, difficulty breathing, or nausea. Risks of the CT scan include the same possible reactions to the intravenous dye as in the IVP (see above).

The CT scanner looks like a tube, and the patient's body enters the center of the tube. Within the tube, a thin, precise beam of x-rays is sent through the patient. A small portion of the beam is absorbed by the patient. Detectors within the tube catch the unabsorbed portion of each x-ray beam and send information back to a fast computer. The computer then combines all of the x-ray information and produces picture images. The most commonly used picture reconstructions show the body in sections, like slices of bread. Radiologists examine the CT pictures carefully, looking for areas where the cancer has spread and for areas of blockage of the kidneys or bladder.

Magnetic Resonance Imaging

Magnetic resonance imaging is the newest and most advanced way to evaluate the interior of the body without surgery. As with ultrasound, there are no known harmful effects of MRI to the body. However, the test does take longer than ultrasound, and it is somewhat more inconvenient for patients. This inconvenience is a trade-off for high-quality images of the bladder and better ability to identify the location of tumors. Patients who are allergic to the dye used for IVP or CT scans typically get an MRI instead.

MRI involves patients entering a small tube, which is actually an array of very powerful magnets. Because of the magnetism, patients are asked to remove all metal objects, such as watches or hair clips, before entering the MR room. Inside the magnetic tube, patients hear loud banging noises when the MR machine begins to take pictures. This noise is normal and is part of how the MRI works. When the MR machine is taking pictures, it is actually "broadcasting" radio signals into the body. After broadcasting this radio signal, the scanner pauses for a fraction of a second. During this time, the patient's body "broadcasts" a signal back to the MR machine. This signal from the body is very much like a short-wave radio signal. The MR machine has powerful computers, which are used to assemble the small radio signals from the patient's body to form a picture.

If you are scheduled for MRI examination, it is a good idea to arrive fifteen to thirty minutes before your actual appointment time. As with other procedures, you will be asked to fill out some forms before you can have an MRI scan. Specifically, these forms are to make sure that you do not have a medical condition that would make it dangerous for you to be in a powerful magnetic field. Some of the more important conditions are listed below:

1. Aneurysm clip: Patients with brain aneurysm clips can only have an MRI if they know the exact type and brand of aneurysm clip. The

MRI technologist will check to make sure that this aneurysm clip is not attracted to the magnetic field.

2. Cardiac pacemaker: No one with a pacemaker should have an MRI. Pacemakers are sensitive electronic devices, and they would be damaged by the powerful MRI magnet.

3. Implanted electrical simulators or pumps: These devices also can be damaged by the magnetic field.

4. Metal in the eye: Patients who have had a prior accident that left metal in an eye should not have an MRI. Since this metal could be affected by the powerful MRI magnet, it could potentially damage the eye.

5. Metal or machine workers: People who grind metal parts as part of their job or who may have been exposed to metal filings should discuss their job with the MRI technologist. There could be a small fragment of metal in the eye which no one knows about. People whose current or past job involves metal filings will have to have an x-ray of the eyes before having an MRI test.

6. Pregnancy: Women who are pregnant in the first trimester should not have an MRI. There is no known injury to the baby, but doctors feel it is better not to have an MRI during this period of fetal development. However, if some sort of imaging is necessary, an MRI is safer than a CT scan, which involves radiation.

After discussing these conditions with you, the MR technologist will have you put on a gown so that zippers or metal snaps on your clothing will not interfere with the MR pictures. You will remove all metal objects from your body, as well as your credit cards and wallet—the magnetic strip on your credit cards would be erased by the MR scanner.

For the procedure, you will lie on your back on a table. After placing several pads on your body, the technologist will advance you into a long, narrow, dark tube. Some patients who have claustrophobia, a fear of small, enclosed spaces, may find this aspect of the MRI very uncomfortable. Therefore, patients should discuss claustrophobia with the MR technologist or their physician ahead of time. Patients who are fearful of small spaces can take a very small dose of a medication such as Valium (5–10

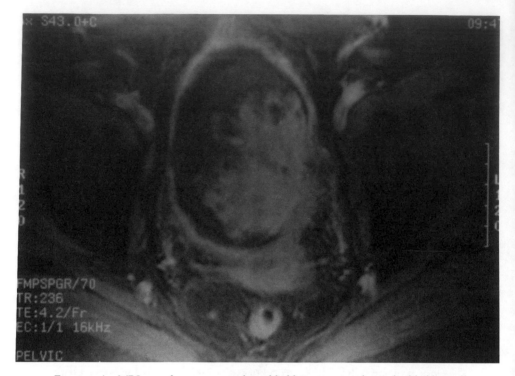

Fig. 3.3. An MRI scan demonstrates a large bladder tumor involving the bladder wall in the patient depicted in this study. The bladder is visible as the oval object in the center; the white tumor material grows out of the bladder wall like a bloom and appears to obstruct most of the bladder's interior.

mg) or Xanax (1–2 mg) beforehand. Valium removes the feeling of claustrophobia in most patients. If your doctor prescribes this medicine for you, make sure someone drives you to the MRI facility and can drive you home after the MRI test. Some patients find that their anxiety about the confined space of the MR machine is alleviated if they close their eyes or wear an eye shade, or blindfold, which the technologist can provide.

Before starting the MR test, soft pads are often placed both under the pelvis and on the front of the patient, over the bladder. This soft pad helps get good pictures of the bladder and close-up views of any abnormalities or tumors. Many MR facilities also give patients a small intramuscular injection in the arm. This injection stops the bowels from moving for about twenty minutes. When the bowels are stationary, the MR pictures look sharper and are more clear.

Finally, a small intravenous catheter may be inserted into a vein in order to inject a dye or contrast agent. This contrast agent is extremely safe, and only a small amount (less than an ounce) is typically injected. About one in forty patients may have a metallic taste from the injection, but most patients only feel a slight coolness in their arm during the injection.

During the MRI test, you will be able to speak to the MR technologist through a microphone. The technologist monitors whatever you say, in case you have any questions. Also, patients usually wear earplugs or head-phones with music, to decrease the noise of the MR scanner. Before your MRI, you can call the facility to find out if you can bring your favorite cassette tape or compact disc to listen to during the MRI test.

In the past few years, there have been an increasing number of advertisements for "open" MRI facilities, which do not make patients feel as if they are enclosed in a tube during the MRI scan. These open MRI scanners are also quieter than traditional MRI scanners because they have less powerful magnets. However, there is a major drawback for patients with bladder cancer; images take up to twice as long to obtain and have lower resolution (they are less clear). At this time, we do not recommend open MRI for our patients with bladder cancer unless the MRI is to examine the brain or spine. In the future, there will probably be improvements in all MRI scanners which will make the test more comfortable.

Which Imaging Test Should I Have?

We have discussed a number of imaging tests that are available for you and your doctor to evaluate your bladder and kidneys. Each test can tell us certain things, and what type of test you should have depends on your medical history. Your doctors will make specific recommendations based on your symptoms. Each imaging test has its advantages.

The IVP examination is often one of the first imaging tests a patient may receive for problems related to the bladder and kidneys. It is relatively inexpensive and quick and provides a good evaluation of the ureters, the tubes that drain urine from the kidneys to the bladder, as well as the kidneys. However, it can detect only relatively large bladder tumors. Ultrasound provides somewhat more information than the IVP, but it cannot see tumors in the ureters. After the ultrasound has detected problems with the kidneys or bladder, a CT scan or MRI is then useful to further define the problem.

For patients with bladder tumors, CT and MRI scans are very useful for seeing inside the body, as both examinations provide a comprehensive view of the internal organs. CT scanning is quicker and more comfortable for the patient. It has the disadvantage of utilizing a dye injection, to which some people are allergic. MRI is particularly good at providing fine detail about the relationship of the bladder tumor to the surrounding organs. This detail may be needed by your doctor, especially if you are being considered for surgery or if the other imaging tests have been contradictory or incomplete.

The most recent advances for patients with bladder tumors have been developed in CT and MR scanning. The newest types of CT scanners are called either "helical" or "spiral" CT scanners. These CT scanners are extremely rapid and provide more detail than older CT scanners. The older scanners take pictures of the body that are oriented like individual slices of a loaf of bread; there is a gap, or space, between each slice, where no pictures are taken. This gap is relatively small (less than half an inch), but it still represents unpictured areas of the body. Spiral or helical CT eliminates this gap. The pictures are also taken about five times faster than with older CT scanners.

MRI scanners are constantly being improved to provide faster, higher-resolution images. Some MRI scanners have "phased array" capability, meaning that higher-resolution, clearer pictures of the inside of the body can be taken. You can ask the radiologist at your MRI facility if this capability is available for bladder imaging. They are as safe as normal MRI, and for you there would be no noticeable difference in the type of MRI. However, your doctors will see pictures that provide more detail.

A recent development for MR imaging is the use of dyes or contrast agents that improve the detection of cancer. One such contrast agent is being developed for looking at lymph nodes. The human body contains many lymph nodes, and they occasionally grow in size without containing

Table 3.3 Screening and Diagnostic Tests for Bladder Cancer

Test	Examines	Discomfort involved
Urinalysis	Urine, looks for blood/ infection	None
Cystoscopy	Tumor in bladder	Mild
IVP	Kidneys and ureters	Mild
US	Kidneys and bladder	None
CT/MRI	Chest/abdomen and pelvis, looks for metastases	Claustrophobia/possible allergy to dye

cancer. However, when bladder cancer spreads to lymph nodes, it also causes the nodes to enlarge. A new contrast agent for MRI that detects whether the enlarged lymph node contains tumor cells is being tested for bladder cancer patients. It will be several years before doctors and researchers have determined its effectiveness for patients with bladder cancer. If successful, this contrast agent will be helpful in telling doctors which lymph nodes to biopsy, or it may indicate that a biopsy is not necessary.

Armed with a knowledge of the types of tests and evaluations that are initially used to discover and characterize bladder cancers, we are prepared to move on to the realm of treatment. As we have seen, most bladder tumors are superficial. This means they are suitable for endoscopic removal, that is, removal using a specialized cystoscope. In the next chapter we explain more about having bladder tumors removed with modern instruments that make surgery without incisions a reality. In addition, we detail the standard treatment for patients who have recurring bladder tumors.

CHAPTER FOUR

Surgery without an Incision

Most of us think surgery must involve cutting through the skin, but that's not always the case. Thanks to the labors of many generations of lens makers and telescope manufacturers, people living at the end of the twentieth century enjoyed an unprecedented opportunity to have surgical procedures of great complexity performed without an incision through the skin. This technique is called *endoscopy*, and the tools used in the technique are called *endoscopes*: small telescopes with versatile operating modifications. Urology is one of the many medical specialties that takes advantage of endoscopic surgery as a viable alternative to so-called open surgery, which is performed through an incision.

The urinary tract was one of the first systems in which scopes outfitted with electric bulbs were used both for routine diagnostic purposes and for surgery. With the development of fiberoptic lens systems and scopes that bend and flex into multiple positions to accommodate the angles of the urinary tract, modern urologic endoscopic surgery can now handle very complex diagnostic and therapeutic challenges. This includes the removal of tumors from the inside of the ureter and the renal pelvis and the routine removal of most bladder tumors. In this chapter, we explain exactly what your urologist is doing when he or she looks into your urinary tract with an endoscope, the benefits of some of the procedures that can be performed with an endoscope, and the associated risks of these procedures.

Cystoscopy

In the previous chapter we looked at the important role the cystoscope plays in diagnosing bladder cancer. Let's look now at the therapeutic function of the cystoscope—how it is used to go beyond diagnosis to treat disease.

The development of powerful light sources for the cystoscope prompted the development of longer and narrower instruments, which could easily reach into the interior of the bladder. With this longer reach and increased versatility, inspection ability was enhanced and surgical procedures such as the biopsy of tumors and the removal of stones became possible without an incision. As noted in chapter 2, a rigid scope is used for operating in the lower urinary tract, but flexible scopes, a significant advance in endoscopy with the advent of fiberoptics, make it possible to carry out complex procedures in the upper urinary tract.

Most modern cystoscopes are equipped with channels that permit small instruments to be passed into the bladder for the purpose of removing tissue, stopping bleeding with a special electrical device called an *electrocautery*, or even performing laser treatment. In addition, instruments can be passed through cystoscopes into the ureters to evaluate the upper urinary tract (these types of studies are usually performed in the operating room with the patient under anesthesia). An illustration of some equipment that your urologist may use during the initial evaluation of your bladder appears in Figure 4.1.

In chapter 3 we explained what you can expect from a diagnostic cystoscopic exam. During this exam, once the scope is inside the bladder, the urologist will examine all of the surfaces of the interior of the organ to see if there are any abnormalities, beginning with the general appearance of the lining of the bladder. Though the tissue is vascular (containing blood vessels), it should not appear red or have abnormally bulging contours. The blood vessels in the lining of the bladder are regularly spaced and of similar size. Irregular or "heaped-up" blood vessels may signal the work of tumor cells, which sometimes secrete substances that induce the growth

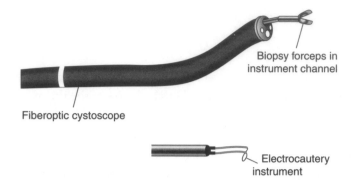

Fig. 4.1. A magnified schematic representation of a flexible cystoscope with biopsy forceps emerging from the end of the scope. The small electrocautery element depicted is used to scrape tumors out of the interior of the bladder and to take samples of the bladder wall.

of a new blood supply for the tumor, a process known as *angiogenesis*. The walls of the bladder are also examined. They should be regular and smooth. Although in many people the bulging of muscle fibers forming the bladder wall are visible through the lining of the bladder interior, this bulging should be more or less uniform.

The connection between the bladder and the ureters are also examined by the doctor performing cystoscopy. These openings—referred to as the ureteral orifices (*orifice* simply means *opening* in Latin)—can assume various shapes but are generally slitlike, delicate, and easy to see because they are located near the bladder neck, just where the urethra and the bladder join. If a ureteral orifice is affected by the growth of a tumor, the opening may be difficult to see. The growth of a tumor is not the only process that can change the appearance of a ureteral orifice. Stones formed in the kidney must pass through the ureter before they can be expelled from the bladder with the urine. Some stones will cause the ureteral orifice to swell (a process known as *edema formation*).

The interior of the prostate is not truly visible during cystoscopy, although the portion of the urethra that runs through the prostate is easily seen during this examination.

If the urologist identifies an abnormality, he or she may elect to biopsy the abnormal-looking area in the office during cystoscopy. A biopsy involves removing a small amount of tissue from the patient using specialized instruments. The most common form of outpatient bladder biopsy is performed with a small pair of grasping forceps that look like a tiny clam shell. The forceps are passed through the interior of the cystoscope into the bladder, and a small portion of the tissue in question is grasped. With a swift pull, a portion of the tissue is detached from the bladder, withdrawn through the scope, and sent to the pathology laboratory for evaluation. Since bladder tumors can be single or multiple, your doctor will pay close attention as he or she inspects the bladder to make sure that every lesion is documented and biopsied if necessary.

Most patients describe a pulling or pinching sensation when a biopsy is taken, although the sensation is brief. Once the biopsy has been obtained, the site where the tissue was removed from the bladder will almost invariably produce a small amount of blood. Although many biopsy

> The procedure was over in less than a half hour. I didn't have any pain, but afterwards there were blood clots when I urinated.

sites would stop bleeding on their own, most urologists feel that bleeding points in the bladder should be controlled at the time the biopsy is taken, to ensure that further bleeding does not occur and cause difficulties like urinary obstruction.

The usual procedure to control biopsy site bleeding is *electrocauterization*; it involves inserting a small wire through the cystoscope and passing electric current through the wire. When the wire is brought into contact with the bleeding tissue, the tissue is singed and the bleeding vessels close and stop bleeding. The sensation of having a biopsy site cauterized in this manner is similar to that of having a cavity treated with a high-speed drill. The pain is brief and tolerable, although some patients complain of either cramping or burning sensations. The discomfort is temporary, and a small number of patients do not feel the biopsy or the cauterization of the biopsy site at all.

Because biopsy of the bladder can cause bleeding, there are certain medicines you should not take before a cystoscopic examination that may

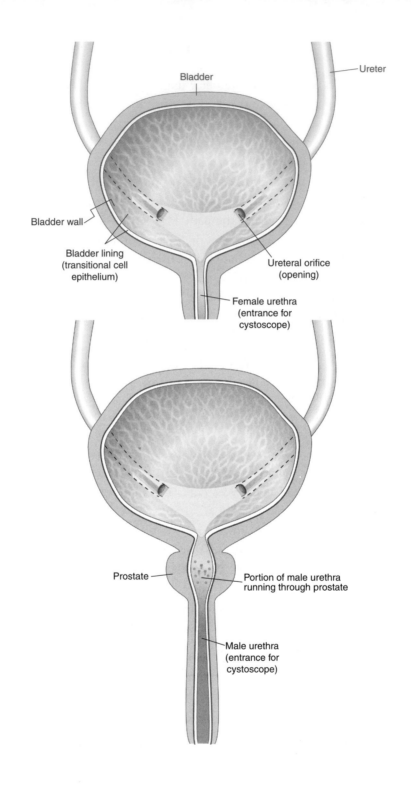

Bladder

Ureter

Bladder wall

Bladder lining
(transitional cell
epithelium)

Ureteral orifice
(opening)

Female urethra
(entrance for
cystoscope)

Prostate

Portion of male urethra
running through prostate

Male urethra
(entrance for
cystoscope)

include biopsy. Your doctor will probably advise you about which medications to avoid before your examination. The following medications could complicate your cystoscopic exam and biopsy, and therefore *should not be taken before cystoscopy:* aspirin, coumadin, nonsteroidal anti-inflammatory medications, and blood thinnners. Tell your doctor if you are taking any of these medications.

After Cystoscopy—What to Expect

Patients generally go home after cystoscopy without much inconvenience. Only rarely do problems arise as a consequence of routine cystoscopy, and they are usually not serious, although some require additional medical attention. Probably the most common symptom patients have after cystoscopy is irritation upon urination and the passage of a small amount of blood in the urine. Since many patients who come to the attention of a urologist have had blood in their urine before, this in itself is not usually terribly upsetting. However, if a patient, particularly one who has had a biopsy, experiences excessive bleeding, the urologist should be notified.

Excessive bleeding is a relative term that should be explained to you in advance by your urologist so that, if it occurs, you will recognize it. The color of urine is often likened to various types of wine. Urine that is barely pink and through which you can clearly see is sometimes compared to blush wine. Slightly darker hued but otherwise clear urine is called rosé, while dark urine is characterized as burgundy colored. Urine can be reddened by a very small quantity of blood in a rather large volume of urine. Consequently, what looks bad to you may seem inconsequential to your physician. We tell patients that if their urine looks like tomato juice, we need to hear from them. Similarly, one urologist we know used to tell patients that if they could not read the daily paper through their urine, they should call him.

FACING PAGE:
Fig. 4.2. Interior views of the female (*top*) and the male (*bottom*) bladder. The ureters enter the bladder on its back side, close to the region where the urethra and bladder meet.

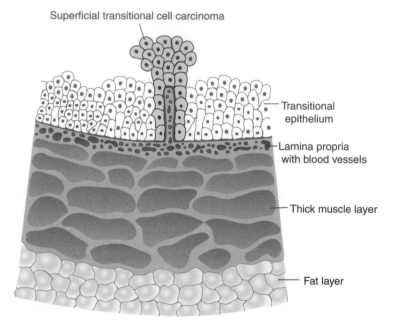

Superficial transitional cell carcinoma

Transitional epithelium

Lamina propria with blood vessels

Thick muscle layer

Fat layer

Fig. 4.3. A schematic representation of a bladder cancer arising from the lining of the bladder, not penetrating the wall of the bladder.

About 5 percent of people who undergo cystoscopy have fever and chills after the procedure. Though all cystoscopic equipment is sterilized before use, it is impossible to sterilize the inside of the human urethra, which always has a few bacteria growing in it. Consequently, it is always possible to get a urinary tract infection after cystoscopy. Many urologists routinely prescribe antibiotics for patients who have had an exam. This is to prevent the development of a symptomatic urinary tract infection that might otherwise require intravenous antibiotics if not treated quickly. The signs and symptoms of a urinary tract infection are:

—fever
—chills
—back pain
—frequent urination
—pain on urination

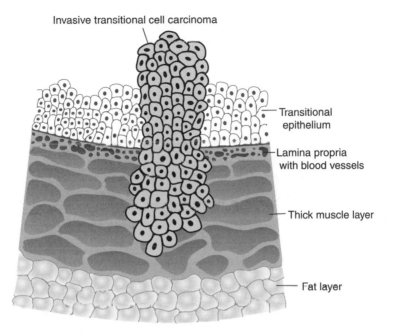

Invasive transitional cell carcinoma

Transitional epithelium

Lamina propria with blood vessels

Thick muscle layer

Fat layer

Fig. 4.4. A schematic representation of a muscle-invasive carcinoma arising from the lining of the bladder and extending both into the bladder and into the muscular layers of the bladder wall.

If you develop any of these symptoms after an exam, contact your urologist.

Let's assume that you've had a cystoscopic examination and your doctor has found something in the bladder that he or she considers abnormal and worthy of further investigation. If a biopsy was performed during cystoscopy, as described above, the next step will be to wait for the pathology report to come back so that you and your physician will know what you are dealing with. The turnaround time for results of biopsies and analysis of other specimens taken at the time of cystoscopy varies, depending upon the doctor's office and the pathology laboratory your doctor works with. At our hospital, it usually takes about five working days to get results of tissue studies back from the lab. Patients are asked to call the office about a week after the procedure to see if there are results that we will need to discuss.

The possible options in patients with potential bladder tumors are limited. If your doctor looks in and sees one lesion, this abnormality is either going to be a superficial bladder tumor or an invasive bladder tumor. The former, as we have seen, is more common, less dangerous, and relatively easy to treat. (Figure 4.3 illustrates what a superficial bladder tumor looks like.) The management of an invasive lesion that has started to grow into the wall of the bladder itself can be complex and will be discussed in detail in the following chapter. (An invasive tumor is shown in Figure 4.4).

A third type of bladder tumor, called *carcinoma in situ* (CIS), also can be discovered during cystoscopy. CIS is still a superficial bladder cancer, but it is an aggressive form. CIS lesions often are described as looking like red velvety patches within the bladder lining. It is important for your urologist to identify these lesions because, although superficial, they are potentially dangerous. CIS lesions are associated with a high rate of relapse and a distinctly higher than average rate of progression than those for other types of superficial tumors.

TURBT—First-Line Surgery

Once the pathologist has evaluated the biopsy and your doctor has interpreted the material, he or she will probably recommend further treatment of the bladder tumor. The first step in the case of superficial lesions not associated with CIS or invasive cancer is complete removal of the tumor or tumors by a process called *transurethral resection of the bladder tumor* (TURBT). In the case of lesions associated with CIS, additional therapy after TURBT will probably be prescribed. A "TUR," as the procedure is generically known among urologists, is an endoscopic or "scope" procedure that does not involve making an incision in the body. The entire removal of a bladder tumor, even a very large tumor, can be accomplished by using an operating scope called a *resectoscope*, which is passed through the urethra into the bladder. *Resect* means to remove a part or all of an organ or structure.

Transurethral surgery is not new, and the tools for this operation have not changed much in the last twenty-five years. The advantage of this approach is clear: it avoids making an incision in the patient's abdomen to remove the cancer. For a TUR, a small, electrified, semicircular loop of wire attached to a trigger mechanism on the scope is moved back and forth through the tumor tissue under direct observation through the scope. There are two ways of viewing the procedure: either the operating surgeon looks through the lens of the scope as he or she resects the tumor, or the scope is attached to a television monitor so the procedure can be viewed by the entire operating team as the resection is done.

Electricity is the force that removes the tumor. As a controlled form of powerful energy, electricity is routinely used in the operating room both to cut tissue and, as we saw in the discussion of biopsy, to stop bleeding after the tissue has been cut. Slices of tumor are removed with each passage of the electrified wire loop, and eventually the entire tumor is separated from the bladder wall. Most superficial bladder tumors are attached to the bladder by a thin stalk of tissue, which can be easily removed using the electric loop. Sometimes the attachment is broader, in which case the removal of the base of the tumor is more challenging. Experienced resectionists can remove most tumors without a great deal of difficulty, though.

Because electricity makes the bleeding vessels contract and seal-off, electrocauterization (or *fulguration*, as it is sometimes called) is extremely useful in scope surgery. The operating surgeon cannot "reach in to the bladder" through the scope and stop bleeding using a sponge or pressure, after all.

The precise removal of bladder tumors with scopes is a specialized form of surgery that is fundamental to the care of bladder cancer patients. It can be performed on an outpatient basis repeatedly, if necessary, with minimal risk to the patient and with generally excellent results. Transurethral surgery is usually performed with the assistance of anesthesia. Whether this is spinal or general is largely a matter of individual surgeon and anesthesiologist preference. Some patients prefer being asleep during surgical procedures, whereas others like to stay awake so that they can talk to the surgical team during the procedure if necessary. There are risks associated with any form of surgery, and endoscopic urologic surgery, while safe, is no exception. A list of the risks associated with TUR appears in Table 4.1. Some of these are obvious and self-explanatory, but others require comment.

Table 4.1 Potential Risks of TUR

Infection	<10%
Injury to bladder	<10%
Bleeding	common
Pain/burning on urination	common
Need to wear catheter afterward for a few days	uncommon

Complications of surgery are always a source of concern for patients and their doctors. One of the fundamental axioms of medicine is to do no harm to the patient. Surgeons and other members of the surgical team take every measure possible to avoid technical problems or mishaps during an operation. But even with the best preventive measures and most competent surgeons, sometimes problems of a technical nature will develop during the course of a procedure.

The most common technical problem that arises during bladder tumor removal by TUR is the unintended perforation of the bladder wall. Usually this is not as serious as it may sound. Most perforations are fairly harmless because the hole in the wall is small and closes spontaneously in a few days. Typically, no long-term adverse consequences result from such small mishaps. Perforations can occur either because the surgeon, in an effort to completely remove all traces of the tumor, digs a bit too deeply into the bladder wall and the electricity produces a deeper bite than was intended, or because the electricity stimulates nerves near the bladder and causes contraction of muscles in the leg. The leg on the side of the bladder that is being worked on may actually "jump," causing the bladder to move while the surgeon is cutting. Such reflex reactions are responsible for a number of bladder injuries each year. Again, these holes do not usually require more than a day or two of urinary catheter drainage to permit the hole in the bladder wall to close.

Some holes in the bladder will not close on their own, however. These may require surgical opening of the lower part of the abdomen to sew up the hole. This is necessary when it appears that the damage to the bladder is sufficient to make more conservative measures risky to the patient's general health. These health risks include infection caused by urine leaking out of the hole in the bladder into the abdominal cavity or problems with normal bodily functions such as digestion.

While the likelihood of injury to the bladder requiring open surgery during TUR is small, there is a fairly high risk of bleeding afterward. In fact, most people see some blood in their urine for a day or two after a bladder tumor is removed. The amount of blood may be small, making the urine barely turn pink, but some blood does leak from the operative site into the urine and is evacuated during every urination. Some patients experience more significant bleeding, and the urine may seem dark red or frankly "bloody." In the case of very bloody urine, we usually recommend that the patient call the office during the day or come to the emergency room if it happens after normal working hours. The reason for seeking medical attention in this circumstance is that blood can accumulate in the bladder, expanding it and actually worsening the bleeding from the site of the tumor removal. It's easy to understand how this happens: blood fills the bladder with clotted material that will not easily pass through the urethra; pressure from the expanding blood clot stretches the walls of the bladder and keeps the bleeding ends of surgically cut blood vessels from contracting and clotting off as they normally would if the bladder were empty; the open blood vessels continue to add blood and more clotting forms, producing a vicious cycle of bladder distention and bleeding.

The remedy for this situation is simple. If a patient has significant bleeding after a TUR, a urinary catheter is placed into the bladder and the bladder is irrigated with sterile saltwater solution. This will remove the clot and stop the bleeding. When large tumors are removed by TUR, some urologists leave a catheter in the patient's bladder for a day or two to ensure that bleeding, clot formation, and overdistention of the bladder do not occur.

Recently, urologic surgeons have incorporated different types of lasers into practice, and these can be very useful in the treatment of some forms of superficial bladder cancer. Lasers, like electricity, are a form of energy that can be harnessed to destroy tumor tissue. Lasers can do this with minimal bleeding or pain and are ideal for the treatment of small, recurrent, low-grade, superficial tumors, either in the office or in the outpatient setting.

What to Expect after TUR

If the tumor that your doctor has discovered is superficial, it is possible that by simply removing the tumor, your problem will be solved—at least for the short term. One of the most troublesome facts doctors and patients face about superficial bladder cancer is that although superficial lesions are rarely life threatening, many recur, even years after the initial diagnosis and apparently successful treatment of the primary (or "presenting") tumor. Some people are lucky and have only one recurrence, while others have multiple recurrences over their lifetime. Up to 70 percent of people with superficial bladder cancer experience a recurrence at some time during their life, but only about 10 to 15 percent of people with superficial bladder cancer develop a more life-threatening form of bladder cancer later in life.

Once the tumor has been removed, your physician will send the specimen for analysis in the pathology laboratory. It usually takes about four days for the pathologists to review the biopsy. Once they have written the final report and your doctor has been informed of the results, he or she will undoubtedly want to review this material with you.

If the tumor is found to have been superficial, solitary, and low grade, your doctor will probably elect to follow your condition closely, conducting surveillance examinations of the bladder every three months for a year or two, then every six months for a year or two, and once a year thereafter. If the tumor is intermediate or high grade, is associated with CIS, or has features that suggest invasion of the superficial layer of the bladder wall but not the muscle (that is, lamina propria invasion, stage T_1—see Table 3.2), then your doctor will probably suggest one of two courses of action, depending upon a variety of individual characteristics of your case. Some surgeons recommend immediate bladder removal for high-grade (3/3) lesions associated with lamina propria invasion or CIS. The reason is that patients with these types of bladder cancers have been found to have high rates of tumor recurrence and progression to more advanced disease that sometimes cannot be cured even when more extensive surgery is performed later. Bladder removal surgery is discussed in greater detail in chapter 5. In recent years an alternative to bladder removal surgery has been developed—the use of drugs that can actually be put directly into the bladder.

Intravesical Drug Therapy

An alternative strategy for superficial bladder cancer treatment has devel·oped with the use of several different types of medical therapies that can be placed directly into the bladder. This is referred to as *intravesical* (*in the bladder*) chemotherapy or immunotherapy. A number of drugs are placed in the bladder after bladder cancer removal in an attempt to minimize the risk of tumor recurrence and progression. These drugs come from a wide variety of sources. It is helpful to know something about these drugs, because they are commonly used and each has its own track record, risks, and benefits. In this section we will explain when and how these drugs are administered, and in the next sections we will discuss the specific drugs that are used and the benefits and risks of each.

Drug therapy after TUR is commonly prescribed for patients with tumors that are:

—large (bigger than 5 cm)
—multiple
—associated with CIS
—high grade and stage (grade 2–3 or stage T_1)

Tumors falling into any of these categories have a higher rate of recurrence and progression than solitary Ta lesions of lower grade or smaller size. The method of drug delivery and the schedule of drug administration are similar for most pharmaceutical agents used in modern doctors' offices. Drug treatment is usually started about two to three weeks after TUR. Patients are asked to limit their fluid intake for about six to twelve hours before coming for the drug treatment to minimize the amount of urine present while the drug is acting on the bladder lining, thus minimizing the likelihood that the drug will be diluted.

We ask all patients who come in for drug treatment after TUR to supply us with a urine sample in the office so we can check for signs of infection before administering the drug. Someone with an active urinary tract infection may have cracks and breaks in the lining of the bladder, which would allow a large amount of the drug placed in the bladder to be absorbed into the person's bloodstream. Such absorption can be harmful to the patient's general health.

If the urine specimen shows no sign of infection, a catheter is placed in the bladder through the urethra and the prescribed drug is infused into the bladder. The patient is asked to avoid urinating for up to two hours so that the solution will be held in the bladder and have adequate time to act on the bladder lining. After the patient urinates, he or she may resume normal activities. About 50 to 70 percent of patients have very good responses to intravesical therapy.

> The doctor told me it was possible that my cancer could be cured with a direct shot of chemotherapy into the bladder. I did that for six weeks, once a week, and had no side effects. After the treatment, I felt like a new man. Prior to that, I had been urinating every 15 minutes.

Most intravesical therapy is given on an outpatient basis. While being catheterized is not pleasant, it involves fairly minimal discomfort and most patients tolerate the therapy without significant difficulty. As noted above, the different drugs used for intravesical therapy after TUR have specific side effects and some risks associated with their use. These are detailed below.

Most chemicals used to treat the inside of the bladder today have been added to the medical armamentarium in the last quarter-century. The most commonly used agents today are:

—Mitomycin C. This is an anticancer drug that has been found to be particularly useful in the treatment of superficial bladder cancer.
—Bacille Calmette-Guerin (BCG). This compound was first introduced into urologic practice in the mid-1970s. It acts as a form of immunotherapy. BCG is one of the most effective agents in the treatment of superficial bladder cancer, although doctors do not fully understand how this drug kills bladder cancer cells.

Mitomycin C

Mitomycin C is converted into a chemical that disrupts normal DNA functions in cancer cells, killing them. One of the major advantages of mitomycin C is that the drug is a relatively large molecule, so it is not easily absorbed through the lining of the bladder into the bloodstream. This means there is only a small risk that the drug will cause the serious side effects (such as suppression of the normal bone marrow's production of blood cells) that could result if the drug were administered intravenously.

Mitomycin C appears to be effective in preventing recurrences in about 50 percent of people who receive it after TUR. The drug is well tolerated in most people, but some specific side effects have been associated with its use. In some people, mitomycin C causes *chemical cystitis*, an irritation of the bladder lining that feels much like a urinary tract infection. Pain in the region of the bladder as well as pain on urination occur in up to 40 percent of patients treated with mitomycin C. These symptoms usually get better with time and resolve completely when therapy is stopped. Allergic reactions, such as rashes on the hands, genitals, and other locations, occur in about 10 percent of patients treated with mitomycin C. These also usually disappear when therapy is stopped. Rarely, topical therapy (ointment applied to the skin) for these rashes is necessary.

Bacille Calmette-Guerin: Intravesical Immunotherapy

Immunotherapy sounds very appealing; the notion that the body's own immune system could be harnessed for the purposes of killing cancer cells seems to make sense and be less destructive than having "toxic" drugs pumped into the body. In the 1970s, investigators in Canada found that a drug prepared from a bacterium related to the one that causes human tuberculosis, when instilled into the bladders of patients with superficial bladder cancers, caused the cancers to recur less frequently. The drug, called Bacille Calmette-Guerin, or BCG, is now used worldwide as a method of controlling superficial bladder cancer relapse.

BCG is considered a form of immunotherapy because it seems to work by causing an immune response in the bladder lining to the BCG organism. In patients whose systems are able to mount such an immune response—which could be described as an allergic reaction on the inside of the bladder—the reaction kills cancer cells. BCG has been used in patients with all forms of superficial bladder cancer, including Ta, CIS, and T_1 lesions. The most common indications for the use of BCG are disease characteristics that indicate a poor prognosis for the future—for example, large tumor size (>3–5 cm), multiple tumors, CIS, and T_1 tumors.

BCG, like mitomycin C, is administered through a catheter in a manner similar to that described above. One dose a week is administered for six weeks. After a resting period of about four to six weeks, patients undergo repeated cystoscopy to see if any residual tumor remains in the bladder. Studies show that after taking BCG in the prescribed manner, about 50 percent of patients will not have a recurrence of bladder cancer in the short term. Long-term studies suggest that about 35 percent of patients will remain disease-free.

A recent study found that even in patients who do not achieve a complete eradication of the tumor with the first six weeks of treatment with BCG, an additional six weeks of therapy markedly improved the overall outcomes. Many patients with CIS and T_1 tumors can be successfully treated with TUR and postoperative therapy with BCG, although patients failing to become tumor free after TUR and twelve weeks of BCG probably should have their bladders removed owing to their very high rate of tumor progression and the potential for development of metastatic bladder cancer (cancer that spreads outside the bladder itself to other structures in the body). Some investigators have estimated that up to half of people who fail to become tumor free after six to twelve weeks of BCG are at risk for the rapid development (within a year or two) of aggressive and difficult to control cancer.

Maintenance Therapy

Maintenance therapy with BCG or another drug has become a much-discussed topic in urologic circles in the past few years. The theory behind maintenance therapy is that a little therapy now and then after the initial course of TUR and intravesical therapy can keep the bladder cancer at bay better than a simple six-week course of treatment. Although a variety of studies now suggest that maintenance therapy may be useful in certain circumstances, the more definitive data regarding this approach comes from a study performed by a consortium of universities (Lamm, D. L., et al., "Maintenance Bacillus Calmette-Guerin Immunotherapy for Recurrent Ta, T_1, and Carcinoma in Situ Transitional Cell Carcinoma of the Bladder: Randomized Southwest Oncology Group Study," *Journal of Urology* 163 [April 2000]: 1124) that examined the role of maintenance BCG therapy. The investigators in that study found that BCG administered intermittently for three years following the initial diagnosis and treatment of a superficial bladder tumor decreased the likelihood of recurrence and may even have diminished the likelihood of tumor progression. This is a remarkable finding and one that probably will be considered somewhat controversial for the next few years unless additional studies are conducted and show the same finding. A negative note is that there appears to be some increased risk of toxicity associated with prolonged BCG administration, including increased irritative urination symptoms, fever, bleeding, and inability to complete therapy.

Surveillance after Treatment: Current Practice, New Tests

After the successful treatment of a superficial tumor, patients are asked to stay in touch with their urologist. As we have seen, even though these tumors can almost always be successfully treated, this is a disease that should be closely followed. Since the majority of bladder cancer patients develop bladder cancer recurrences at some time in their lives, it makes sense to catch these recurrences early, before the tumors become very large or have a chance to change character and become aggressive—which happens in about 10 to 15 percent of all patients with superficial disease.

As noted above, the standard method for following patients after bladder tumor therapy is to perform cystoscopy every three months for two years, every six months for two years after that, and then once a year for life. The schedule makes sense because it provides intensive surveillance during the initial two years following the treatment, which is when most relapses occur. However, this schedule is not written in stone. Surveillance patterns seem to have been made up based on our best guesses about recurrence patterns. Your urologist may have a slightly different pattern of follow-up for you, and there is nothing wrong with that as long as both you and the urologist keep a close eye on the long-term problem. Once you have had bladder cancer, you need to view it as a lifelong problem, and both you and your doctor need to reach a comfortable agreement about how best to take care of you as an individual.

The prospect of frequent cystoscopic examinations usually bothers patients. As with many diagnostic procedures, the examination is a bit nerve-racking not so much because of the discomfort but because of the worry associated with the possibility of discovering another tumor. This trepidation on the part of patients has not been lost on doctors or investigators in the pharmaceutical industry. For the past decade, scientists have been working to develop laboratory tests that could replace routine cystoscopic evaluations, and their work is beginning to pay off. In the early 1990s, a series of tests that could detect bladder cancer–related molecules in urine specimens became available. The first to gain FDA approval was the bladder tumor antigen test (BTA for short), marketed by the Bard Company. The BTA test in its current form looks like a home pregnancy kit. A small amount of urine is applied to the test apparatus, and in a matter of minutes, if cancer-related molecules are present, a color change is visible on a test strip. A color change means that bladder cancer could be present and further studies should be performed. Other tests like this one, such as Matritech's NMP-22 test and the new Mentor FDP dipstick test, also detect substances in the urine that have been associated with the presence of bladder cancer cells.

These tests are good but not perfect. All are FDA approved as tests that can be performed in addition to cystoscopy for the detection of recurrent bladder cancer. None of these tests has been approved for use as a replacement for cystoscopy, and none has been approved for use as a means of modifying cystoscopic schedules of surveillance for recurrent bladder cancer. A variety of additional tests are currently being developed to improve the detection of bladder cancers. It is possible that in the future, a simple test of urine at your family doctor's office may suffice for routine bladder cancer surveillance, a development that would please physicians and patients alike.

Superficial bladder cancer is a manageable disease that can be cured outright in some patients and controlled successfully in many more. Superficial bladder cancer resembles other chronic diseases that many people develop as they age. The good news is that the superficial bladder tumor can usually be controlled with limited surgery such as TUR and, when necessary, intravesical chemotherapy or immunotherapy using drugs like BCG and mitomycin C.

The biggest problem in treating superficial bladder cancer is that some people do not respond completely to the currently available therapies and others go on to develop more aggressive tumors during their lifetimes. Although this group is the minority of all people with bladder cancer, they present the greatest challenge to urologists; in contrast to superficial lesions that can be controlled by TUR with or without intravesical therapy, superficial tumors that do not respond to treatment and tumors that either progress to or are first seen as a muscle-invasive cancer can be life-threatening. The approaches to these tumors are described in the following chapters. Since aggressive surgery was the first therapy and remains the gold standard for muscle-invasive tumors, we begin there, in chapter 5.

CHAPTER FIVE

Bladder Removal and Urinary Tract Reconstruction

Approximately 25 percent of people with bladder cancer are first seen by the doctor after the tumor has invaded the muscle wall of the bladder. Only a few of these patients have a previous history of superficial bladder cancer, which makes physicians suspect that invasive bladder cancer is of a different type than the superficial tumors discussed in chapter 4. Muscle-invading bladder cancer has a bad reputation, which is well deserved. Tumors that invade the muscle wall of the bladder have the capability of spreading to other parts of the body with little warning. Once these tumors have spread, treatment and cure become much more difficult. For this reason, urologists have traditionally taken the position that if the tumor has invaded the bladder wall and there is no evidence from x-ray studies that the tumor has spread elsewhere in the body yet, the bladder should be removed completely. Although complete removal of the bladder for the treatment of invasive bladder cancer has been performed for more than a hundred years, the modern era of complete bladder removal surgery did not begin until the middle of the twentieth century.

In this chapter, we describe what is involved in making the decision to offer a patient major bladder cancer surgery, how this type of surgery is performed, and some of the details involved in urinary tract reconstruction following bladder removal. In addition, we will go over the specific details of recovery following bladder cancer surgery of this type, a theme that will be expanded on in chapter 6.

Who Needs Bladder Removal Surgery?

Bladder removal surgery is serious, and the decision to offer a patient this surgery involves making several specific decisions based on information obtained during the clinical evaluation of the patient. The first "rock-solid" indication that a patient may require bladder removal surgery is finding muscle invasion by bladder cancer cells in the biopsy obtained from the patient's tumor. As we have already seen, these biopsies are usually performed with a special scope. Once muscle invasion has been identified, the urologist usually orders a series of CAT scans or an MRI. These tests give the physicians information about whether or not the tumor has spread to other parts of the body or is likely contained within the bladder wall or the tissues just surrounding the bladder. These types of scans are also useful because they give information about whether or not lymph nodes in the region of the bladder are involved. If these scans show no evidence of what is referred to as "distant" disease, the urologist generally recommends either partial or complete removal of the urinary bladder. These types of operations are called *partial* or *complete* (or sometimes *radical*) *cystectomy*.

Partial or complete bladder removal surgery is considered the surest treatment of invasive bladder cancer. This is more or less because, until very recently, no other effective therapy for invasive cancer was available. As we discuss in chapters 7 and 8, some invasive cancers can now be treated with chemotherapy and radiation therapy combinations. However, that approach, which is generically referred to as "bladder sparing," has only recently become widely available and is still considered controversial and, by some, experimental. The precedent was set by surgeons, and consequently most urologists still consider removal of the bladder to be the most effective way to treat an invasive tumor. Although the majority of invasive bladder cancers tend to be large and involve a significant portion of the bladder, about one in twenty tumors is located in such a way that the tumor and a portion of surrounding normal tissue can be removed, preserving the remaining portion of the bladder. This approach, called a *partial cystectomy*, is rarely performed, for the following reasons: Tumors that are amenable to this type of surgery must be small and located in a place in the bladder that is easily accessible to the surgeon, such as the roof or dome. In addition, the remainder of the bladder must be completely free of tumor cells. Such conditions are relatively rare, and consequently most patients are not offered this type of therapy. However, in patients meeting the above criteria, partial cystectomy is very effective and can result in excellent long-term survival and disease control.

More often, the cancer is located in parts of the bladder that are not easily approached using the partial cystectomy technique. Many people have large tumors or have many tumors that are located in more than one place in the bladder. For this type of individual, complete removal of the bladder is the standard recommendation and has the most benefits for the patient.

The benefits of bladder removal surgery are disease control, eradication of symptoms associated with bladder cancer, and long-term survival. The benefits are most likely to apply to people who have cancer that, while invasive, does not extend beyond the bladder wall. Stages T_1 and T_2 bladder cancer have the best long-term survival rates after cystectomy, as can be seen in Figure 5.1, which illustrates the long-term survival of bladder cancer patients treated at Johns Hopkins between 1984 and 1996. As you can see, patients with organ-confined bladder cancer have an excellent prognosis.

Patients with more advanced disease (stages above T_3) have a poorer outcome. Accordingly, some of those patents are now offered chemotherapy to increase their likelihood of survival after surgery.

What If the Tumor Is Outside the Bladder?

Bladder removal surgery is usually not offered to patients whose bladder cancers have spread beyond the bladder. Occasionally, patients who suffer from pelvic pain, significant ongoing bleeding, or other problems related to bladder function that are the direct result of the tumor are offered bladder removal to relieve these symptoms. Patients with advanced bladder cancer who are not bothered by symptoms such as bleeding or irritation are usually treated with chemotherapy with or without radiation therapy. Extensive bladder removal surgery is unlikely to produce a significant change in these patients' overall prognosis and may in fact delay the ad-

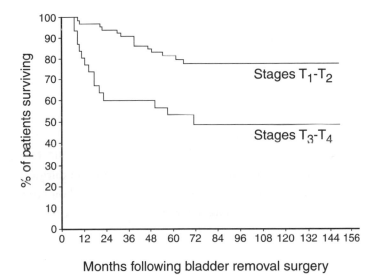

Fig. 5.1. Disease-specific survival of patients with different stage bladder cancer undergoing bladder removal therapy at Johns Hopkins Hospital, followed for a period of at least ten years. Patients with T_1 and T_2 tumor have organ-confined bladder cancer. Patients with T_3 and T_4 bladder carcinoma have tumors extending through the wall and into adjacent structures. Reprinted from Schoenberg et al., "Local Recurrence and Survival Following Nerve Sparing Radical Cystoprostatectomy for Bladder Cancer: Ten-Year Followup," *Journal of Urology* 155: 490–94.

ministration of potentially helpful total-body therapy that can be provided by the intravenous administration of appropriate medications (see chapter 8).

What about Patients with Superficial Cancers?

Some people with superficial bladder cancer are offered bladder removal surgery if all other measures fail to control their tumors. This is an extremely unusual situation these days, since many people with superficial bladder cancer can have their tumors controlled through the use of endoscopic surgical techniques and the administration of specific medicines into the bladder itself, as described in chapter 4. Some superficial tumors do not respond to these measures, however, and people with this condition are offered complete bladder removal and urinary tract reconstruction.

Impact of Bladder Removal on Sexual Function

In men, removal of the bladder also involves removal of the prostate. The prostate is intimately attached to the bladder and can serve as a reservoir for bladder cancer cells if it is not removed. Removal of the prostate results in problems with sexual function after surgery in many men and results in infertility in all cases since the procedure automatically results in interruption of the flow of sperm from the testicle to the urethra during ejaculation. Modifications to the procedure for prostate removal due to prostate cancer have been extended to the performance of complete cystectomy in male patients. The nerves responsible for erections in men are located just behind the prostate and can be preserved through a careful surgical technique developed at Johns Hopkins by Dr. Patrick Walsh in the early 1980s. This highly successful technique has resulted in the preservation of sexual function in many individuals undergoing radical prostatectomy. In 1984, the technique of nerve preservation was extended to complete bladder and prostate removal for patients with bladder carcinoma. Subsequent studies at Johns Hopkins have demonstrated that nerve-sparing cystoprostatectomy can result in preservation of sexual funciton in approximately 60 percent of men age fifty or younger, 50 percent of men age sixty or younger, and 35 percent of men between the ages of sixty and seventy.

In women, the standard operation for bladder removal used to involve complete removal of not just the bladder and urethra but also the uterus, cervix, ovaries, fallopian tubes, and a portion of the vagina. This extensive procedure, known as an *anterior exenteration*, was thought to be useful because bladder cancers in women occasionally invaded the cervix, uterus, or vagina. Recently, studies performed in both the United States and in Europe have shown that bladder cancer, even if invasive, rarely extends to these adjacent organs. Accordingly, bladder removal in women now rarely requires the removal of all of these surrounding structures. This has a profound effect on how women recover from bladder removal surgery (see below).

The impact on sexual function appears to be age specific, with younger men more likely to regain potency (the ability to have an erection satisfactory for sexual relations) if nerve-sparing techniques are employed during bladder removal. Young women, too, recover better than older women. Sexually active people of all ages should discuss sexual recovery after bladder removal surgery with their surgeon before the operation is performed.

Getting Ready for Major Surgery

Once your doctor has told you that you are a candidate for major bladder cancer surgery, you will become involved in the complex process of determining whether or not this type of therapy is appropriate for you and if alternatives exist that could provide you with an equivalent likelihood of cure but which would preserve your bladder. If you have a superficially invasive bladder cancer, such as a type in clinical stage T_{2a} or T_{2b}, an alternative to major bladder removal surgery exists and should be discussed with your doctor. Read more about this in chapter 7.

After you have reviewed this chapter and other information about the surgery, you may decide that bladder removal surgery offers you the best chance of cure, even though there are significant risks associated with this type of therapy. If you choose to proceed with surgery, your doctor will review the risks and the course of therapy with you in great detail. To understand why this type of surgery is complex, why the recovery time after surgery is lengthy, and what the potential hazards are, it is helpful to understand the specifics of bladder removal in some detail. What follows is a description of the preparation for surgery at our hospital, the list of the risks as we understand them for bladder removal surgery and urinary tract reconstruction, and a general time schedule that seems to apply to our patients for both the hospital stay and the home recovery.

Getting ready for bladder removal surgery is similar to the preparation that any patient undergoes in anticipation of a major surgical procedure. Most patients are required to visit their family doctor for a complete preoperative physical examination, which includes certain routine laboratory tests such as an EKG and chest x-ray.

Some patients will elect to donate their own blood prior to surgery to minimize the likelihood that they will require transfusion of blood obtained from someone else. In the era of heightened awareness about

Table 5.1 Potential Risks of Cystectomy

Need for transfusion	<50%
Bleeding	<25%
Bowel obstruction	<10%
Infection	<10%
Injury to other organs	<10%
Blood clots leading to emboli	<5%
Death	<2%
Failure to cure	(depends on stage)

transfusion-related diseases such as HIV and hepatitis, this approach seems sensible, but it can be both inconvenient and sometimes debilitating in elderly patients. It is worth remembering that the risk of contracting HIV from a blood transfusion is now considered to be 1 in two million. The risk of contracting hepatitis is about 1 in 70,000. Since the blood supply is relatively safe, most people do not need to donate their own blood prior to bladder removal surgery, although some will insist upon doing this for their own peace of mind. There is no "right" answer to the question of whether or not you should donate blood. This is a personal matter that you should discuss with your treating physician.

Any patient having a major surgical procedure will meet with the anesthesiologist prior to surgery. It is the job of the anesthesiologist to inform you about different options for complete pain control during surgery. Most patients who undergo bladder removal surgery are given what is referred to as a *general anesthetic*. Some patients, for health reasons, may require spinal anesthesia instead, although this is extremely unusual. If the patient considering bladder removal surgery has many other health problems, a preoperative consultation with staff from the intensive care unit may also be useful, to make sure that special postoperative needs are anticipated.

An important part of your preoperative preparation for major surgery is the opportunity to consult your physician freely prior to the actual day of surgery. You should certainly ask your surgeon any and all questions you may have, so that you will be completely familiar with his or her plans at the time of your operation, as well as with the risks involved in the surgery. In addition, it may be helpful to talk to other patients who have been treated by the same physician or team of physicians and who have had the same procedure that will be performed on you. Most surgeons are very familiar with the operations they offer patients, but they tend to be less familiar with the personal experience of being a patient. It would be quite unusual to come upon a surgeon who has had the surgery that you're going to have. Doctors tend to understand health care from the doctor's perspective. You, as a consumer and a patient, will want to hear about what it is like to be on the receiving end of the health care that is going to be delivered. Talking to other patients who have been in a similar situation is frequently very helpful.

Bladder removal surgery, like many modern operations, requires not only the removal of a problem but also the construction of a solution to the problem that organ removal creates. Once the bladder has been removed, a route for the safe passage of urine from the kidneys to outside the body must be created. If such a passage were not constructed after bladder removal, urine would accumulate inside the body cavity and ultimately result in a patient's death. Patients often ask if an artificial bladder is available to replace the body's natural one after a cystectomy. Although attempts have been made to develop artificial reservoirs, the body does not tolerate the introduction of foreign material into the urinary tract. Anything other than the patient's own tissue can cause the formation of calcium deposits and stones, which ultimately damage the urinary tract. Accordingly, surgeons have spent the last seventy-five years attempting to construct various types of urinary conduits and reservoirs out of segments of the intestinal tract. The small intestine and parts of the large intestine are well-suited for this purpose. Several types of urinary tract reconstructions are commonly offered. Some of the details involved in creating these reconstructions are described below.

Lower Urinary Tract Reconstruction

Ileal Conduit

Although the bladder has been removed, the kidneys and ureters remain, as does the urethra below the level of the prostate in male patients. In female patients, depending upon the extent of surgery, the urethra may also be preserved below the level of its attachment to the bladder neck. The challenge that the surgeon now faces is how to reconstruct the urinary tract in such a way that the urine will be safely conveyed from the body at minimum inconvenience to the patient.

The simplest form of reconstruction, and one that is most commonly employed in the United States today, is called an *ileal conduit*. This form of reconstruction has been routinely performed since the 1950s. A small piece of the *ileum*, a the portion of the small intestine, is disconnected from the remainder of the intestinal tract. One end is closed with sutures and the other end is attached to the skin on the right side of the abdomen. A small *stoma* (the Greek work for *mouth*) is fashioned where the open end of the "conduit" is attached to the skin. A plastic appliance called an ostomy bag is then fitted over the stoma to collect urine that passively drains continuously from the mouth of the ileal conduit. The ureters are implanted into the back of the ileal conduit near the closed end. Figure 5.2 is an illustration of this type of urinary tract reconstruction. Once the conduit has been created, the remaining normal intestinal tract is reconstituted by attaching the ends together to permit the passage of food through the remaining intestines. Once intestinal continuity has been re-established, the patient's abdomen is closed and the operation is over.

The ileal conduit reconstruction is very popular because it is simple to perform and very reliable and has been associated with few long-term complications. Despite this good track record, there are risks and disadvantages of an ileal conduit, which you must be aware of before deciding upon this type of reconstruction. The obvious disadvantage of the ileal conduit is that it requires the patient to wear an ostomy bag for life. Although this seems like a tremendous inconvenience for people who are not accustomed to life with an ostomy, it should be emphasized that an

FACING PAGE:
Fig. 5.2. A schematic representation of the section of bowel used for construction of an ileal conduit (A). An ileal conduit is shown with a stoma exiting on the right side of the patient's abdomen just below the umbilicus (navel). The remaining bowel has been sewn back together to reestablish intestinal continuity (B).

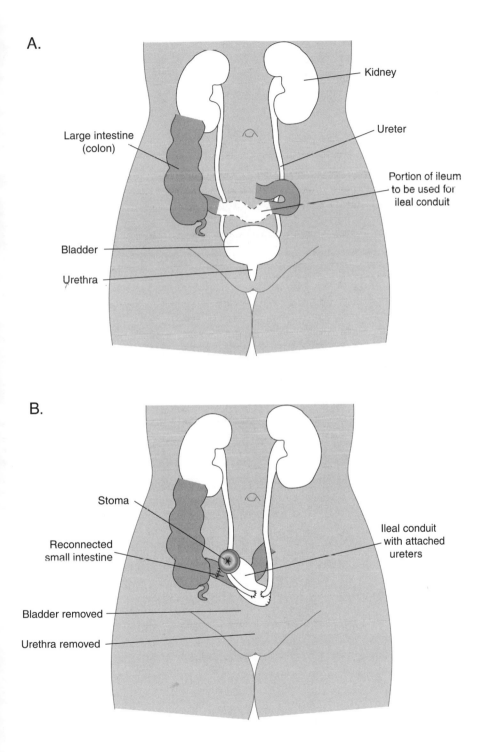

A.

Kidney

Ureter

Portion of ileum
to be used for
ileal conduit

Large intestine
(colon)

Bladder

Urethra

B.

Stoma

Reconnected
small intestine

Ileal conduit
with attached
ureters

Bladder removed

Urethra removed

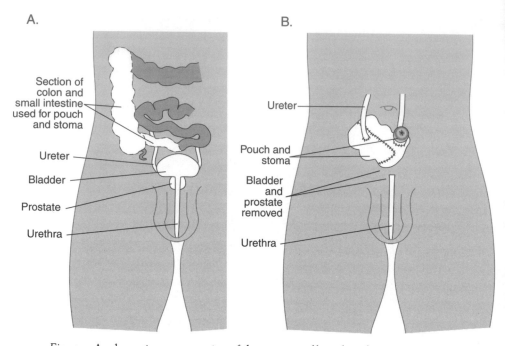

A.

Section of colon and small intestine used for pouch and stoma

Ureter

Bladder

Prostate

Urethra

B.

Ureter

Pouch and stoma

Bladder and prostate removed

Urethra

Fig. 5.3. A schematic representation of the segment of bowel used to create a continent catheterizable reservoir (A). To the right (B), a continent catheterizable reservoir is depicted with the stoma exiting in the midline near the patient's umbilicus (navel). The stoma can be placed in a variety of locations depending upon patient anatomy and surgeon preference. Our preference is to place the stoma in the belly button to make it inconspicuous.

ostomy is compatible with all of the daily activities of normal life, including sexual activity, strenuous physical activity, sports, and recreation. Since the ostomy bag is small and inconspicuous, patients seem to accommodate to a urinary ostomy extremely quickly once they get the hang of applying the ostomy bag to the stoma in the abdominal wall. This takes practice. (You'll learn more about how to take care of a stoma in chapter 6.)

The risks of urinary tract reconstruction apply to almost all forms of surgery designed to reconstitute the urinary tract (see Table 5.2). Whether you choose an ileal conduit or a more complex reconstruction, the immediate postsurgical risks and many of the long-term problems remain the same. Patients with ileal conduits are at immediate risk postoperatively for a series of generic problems associated with major surgery, which include

Table 5.2 Potential Risks of Urinary Tract Reconstruction

Possible need for additional surgery	20%
Scar formation causing blockage of flow, either where ureters are connected or where reconstruction is connected to skin	10–20%
Need to catheterize	<15%
Kidney stone formation	10%
Infection	<10%
Metabolic imbalances	<10%
Failure to empty	<5%
Leakage of urine into the body during healing	<5%

bleeding, infection, bowel obstruction (a postoperative situation in which the intestines temporarily fail to convey their contents in the right direction, leading to abdominal bloating, nausea, and sometimes vomiting), and leakage of urine into the abdominal cavity where the ureters have been attached to the conduit.

Long-term complications of ileal conduit reconstruction include chronic urinary tract infections; slow but steady deterioration of renal function due to kidney stone formation; chronic infection or a process called *reflux*, during which urine excreted by the kidneys into the ileal conduit washes back into the kidneys, disturbing normal renal function; scar formation where the ureters are attached to the ileal conduit, leading to obstruction of urine flow from the kidney into the ileal conduit and subsequent kidney damage; scar formation where the stoma is created at its attachment to the abdominal wall, leading to obstruction of urine flow out of the ileal conduit and subsequent kidney damage; hernia development adjacent to the stoma; and chronic intermittent bowel obstruction. Despite this long list of potential problems, most patients with ileal conduit reconstructions do extremely well.

An Internal Reservoir

When surgeons first began removing the bladder because of disease within this organ, they faced the same challenge that urologists face today—how to provide a safe passage for urine once the principal organ of urine storage and excretion has been removed. Initially, this problem was solved by simply attaching the ureters into the segment of the large intestine adjacent to the rectum. This clever approach allowed the patient to use the colon for urine storage and control the urine flow with the anus when the patient wished to release the accumulated urine that collected in the intestinal tract. This operation, referred to as a *ureterosigmoidostomy*, is still occasionally performed but has fallen out of favor because patients developed significant metabolic abnormalities, some of them quite severe. In addition, older patients with less perfect anal tone were frequently troubled by incontinence.

The goal of creating an alternative internal compartment for the storage of urine has fascinated urologists for much of the century. Almost every segment of the intestinal tract has been used in an attempt to create such a reservoir over the years. International experience suggests that internal reservoirs can be created out of portions of the small intestine, the large intestine, or from combinations of both, with the equivalent functional characteristics. Many individual physicians have devoted their careers to the development of a specific type of internal reservoir. A review of the scientific literature shows that many of these reconstructions bear the names of their creators or the institutions at which these physicians work. Despite the many different names for various reconstructions, these procedures all produce an internal reservoir with a capacity to store urine for approximately four to six hours satisfactorily. Some drawings of various internal reservoirs appear in Figure 5.3.

Initially, when physicians in the 1950s sought to develop reliable internal reservoirs using segments of the large intestine, the reservoir was connected to the outside of the body by a small piece of additional intestinal material that permitted the passage of a catheter into the reservoir in order to empty accumulated urine. This type of reconstruction for the use of a catheter has many variations and is still performed today on patients whose urethra contains cancer cells and must be removed. These reconstructions are also often performed on patients whose normal control mechanism (the sphincter) is not thought to be strong enough to provide adequate urinary continence if the internal reservoir is attached directly to the remaining urethra after bladder removal. For many years, catheteri-

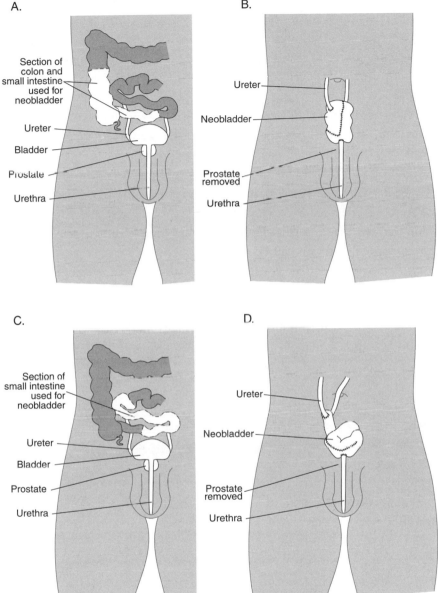

A.

Section of
colon and
small intestine
used for
neobladder

Ureter

Bladder

Prostate

Urethra

B.

Ureter

Neobladder

Prostate
removed

Urethra

C.

Section of
small intestine
used for
neobladder

Ureter

Bladder

Prostate

Urethra

D.

Ureter

Neobladder

Prostate
removed

Urethra

Fig. 5.4. A. The segment of bowel used to create a neobladder. B. A neobladder is constructed and attached to the patient's remaining urethra. C. The segment of bowel used to create an alternate form of neobladder (Studer-type). D. The ureters are attached and a segment of the Studer-type neobladder is connected to the remaining urethral stump to facilitate normal voiding through the urethra.

zable reservoirs were the only form of internal urinary tract reconstruction offered to women, because women undergoing bladder removal for cancer underwent urethra removal as well. Since the recent demonstration that the urethra is infrequently affected by most bladder cancers in women, it is now possible to offer both men and women with disease-free urethras an internal reservoir that is attached directly to the urethra, providing the patient with the ability to urinate more or less normally.

Most urologists consider an internal reservoir connected to the urethra to be the form of urinary tract reconstruction most closely approximating the "normal" configuration of the urinary tract. Accordingly, and not surprisingly, most physicians consider this the ideal form of urinary tract reconstruction, as long as it can be performed safely in the motivated patient. Any internal reservoir attached to the urethra is often referred to by urologists as a *neobladder*, using the Latin word for *new*.

Internal reservoirs that permit the reasonable approximation of normal urinating postoperatively or utilize a catheterizable mechanism seem like a wonderful advance to most patients when they first learn about them. It is certainly true that the development of these types of reconstructions has particularly benefited patients who, for personal reasons, do not wish to consider surgery that includes the creation of external stoma. Nonetheless, complex urinary tract reconstruction is associated with a number of risks and complications, which the patient must be aware of preoperatively in order to make an informed decision about what form of urinary tract reconstruction makes most sense for him or her.

Internal reservoirs that can be catheterized intermittently through a connection with the skin require some form of corrective surgery or intervention 20 percent of the time. Said another way, about one patient in five with a catheterizable internal reservoir will require some form of surgery to "tune-up" the reconstruction and improve its function at some point. In particular, the catheterizable mechanism itself, usually a flap valve that permits the introduction of a catheter to syphon urine out of the reservoir but prevents urine leakage in between catheterizations, often requires some form of corrective surgery later. The success of the initial surgery and the need for follow-up surgery varies from medical center to medical center, but you should keep in mind that scar formation, obstruction of the ureteral connections to the internal reservoir, chronic urinary tract infection, and catheterization mechanism dysfunction all complicate this type of reconstruction and therefore could complicate your recovery.

Similarly, attachment of an internal reservoir to the urethra is also associated with risks and potential complications, the most important of which are urinary incontinence (more common in men than in women, affecting as many as 15 % of men who undergo neobladder reconstruction after cystectomy); the inability to empty the neobladder (which occurs in about 5 % of male patients and as many as 30 to 40 % of female patients), requiring intermittent, potentially lifelong catheterization through the urethra to facilitate adequate drainage of urine from the neobladder; scar formation at the connection of the urethra to the new bladder, resulting in obstruction of urine flow out of the new bladder (a problem that requires minor surgical therapy that can usually be performed with a scope); and other general problems associated with attachment of ureters to pieces of bowel (kidney stone formation, chronic urinary tract infection, and intermittent bowel obstruction).

Generally speaking, the rate of significant complications following complex urinary tract reconstruction is relatively low when the procedure is performed by experienced surgeons. The rate is not zero, however, and you must consider your tolerance for risk and inconvenience as well as your willingness to undergo repair surgery later in life. In this regard, it is particularly helpful talk to patients who have had various forms of urinary tract reconstructions. Although studies done in these populations suggest that patients tend to accommodate to all forms of urinary tract reconstruction well, you may get a sense from talking to the patients themselves as to which type of reconstruction might be most compatible with your expectations, tolerance for risk, and lifestyle.

How Long Does All of This Take?

Many patients want to know how long the process, including surgery and subsequent recuperation, takes. Although everyone is different in this regard, it is possible to draw a general outline. The outline below basically follows the course of a patient at our hospital who undergoes diagnosis, staging consultation, preoperative preparation, bladder removal, urinary tract reconstruction, in-hospital recuperation, and recuperation at home until he or she is able to return to work.

Diagnosis, Staging, and Preoperative Preparation

Most patients with bladder cancer go to a urologist with signs and symptoms suggestive of a problem in the lower urinary tract. An IVP is performed to evaluate the kidneys and ureters, and cystoscopy is performed to evaluate the interior bladder. If a tumor is discovered, a biopsy is performed. From the initial diagnosis to the time that a muscle-invasive tumor is confirmed usually takes one to two weeks. Once muscle invasion has been identified, a CAT scan or MRI scan and, if necessary, a bone scan and other specialized x-rays can be obtained within a few days of diagnosis to complete the staging process. The process of staging provides both the patient and the physician with information about the extent of cancer. Once it has been firmly established that the tumor does not appear to have extended beyond the bladder wall, preparations for surgery can be made.

Usually, it takes about three or four weeks to prepare a patient for major bladder surgery. Most patients undergo preoperative medical testing, and many elect to donate their own blood. In addition, time is invested in conversations with physicians, other patients, and consultants before surgery to ensure the best possible postoperative outcome. Once a patient has chosen to undergo complex urinary tract reconstruction utilizing segments of intestine, specialized x-rays of the intestines or actual examination of the interior of the large intestine using a scope may be necessary to make sure the large intestine does not contain evidence of diseases such as cancer, diverticulosis, or other inflammatory problems that would make using this portion of bowel dangerous in urinary tract reconstruction.

Once cleared for surgery (given approval by their medical doctor), patients take cleansing laxatives and stay on a clear liquid diet for two days prior to surgery to ensure that the intestinal tract is free of contaminating intestinal contents. This "bowel-prep" reduces the likelihood of serious infection after surgery and is almost universally recommended by surgeons who perform these types of operations. Once the patient has been completely prepared for surgery, he or she has a final meeting with the anesthesiologist to confirm the specific type of anesthetic to be used, and then it is time to go to the operating room.

Surgery

Operating rooms vary in appearance from hospital to hospital. Regardless of the room's appearance, similar types of medical professionals—nurses, surgeons, anesthesiologists, surgical assistants—are encountered in an OR. The room is illuminated by bright lights designed to help surgeons see inside the body. The lights can be somewhat dazzling at first. Operating rooms tend to be somewhat cool, too, because the operating team wears heavy gowns and multiple layers of clothing to ensure sterility during surgery. To keep a patient warm during surgery, specially designed heating blankets are applied to portions of the patient's body not involved in the operation.

The operating room is full of equipment, such as a machine designed to administer anesthesia and monitors that the anesthesiologist uses to ensure that the patient is safely asleep throughout the operation. Nurses and surgical assistants set up equipment and instruments and arrange all of the tools necessary for performing the operation. Everyone wears special scrub suits, caps, and masks to help keep the equipment from being contaminated. You are asked to lie down on the operating table and then you are covered with warm blankets. The anesthesiologist administers the sedative to relax you and then lets you drift off to sleep.

Once you are asleep, your body is prepared for surgery. Your gown is removed, and your abdomen and genital area are shaved. Specialized soap designed to kill bacteria is applied to the skin of your abdomen to minimize the risk of infection after surgery. Sterile sheets are then placed all around you, and the operation begins.

The specifics of bladder removal are well known to most urologists, and the details involved in the actual surgical procedure should be familiar to you, so you will be well prepared for the complete experience of undergoing this type of surgery. Once you are asleep and completely prepared for surgery, an incision is made in the lower part of your abdomen. Most surgeons perform this operation through an incision that runs from just below the belly button to the bone above the genitalia. An alternative is to perform the procedure through what is known as a bikini incision, although most surgeons continue to use the more standard approach. The incision is carried down through the layers of the abdominal wall to reveal the internal cavity in which many of the abdominal organs are located—the peritoneum.

The surgical team then removes lymph node material located on either side of the bladder to test for the presence of cancer cells. If spread of the tumor is discovered in the lymph nodes, your surgeon may elect to stop the operation, close the abdomen, and plan on administering chemotherapy before reconsidering additional surgical therapy. This is a point of contention among surgeons, and many doctors will proceed with bladder removal even if a few lymph nodes are shown to have cancer cells in them. This is a point you should probably discuss with your doctor prior to surgery so that you can both agree on a sensible plan should lymph node involvement be identified during a preliminary phase of your operation.

Once the lymph nodes have been removed, attention is turned to removal of the bladder, as well as the removal of the prostate in male patients or, in female patients, the possible removal of the uterus, cervix, and a small portion of the vagina. There are a variety of specific techniques used by surgeons to complete this phase of the operation. The details involved in the preservation of nerves responsible for maintaining sexual function may be a topic you wish to discuss with your physician prior to surgery. If you are contemplating a procedure that involves attachment of a reconstructed bladder to the urethra, you will want to be sure to discuss what will happen if your physician is not able to utilize your urethra, either for anatomic reasons or because of residual cancer discovered in the substance of the urethra at the time of surgery. Your surgeon will doubtless outline the first steps involved in completing your operation for you. Nonetheless, you should feel very free to ask detailed questions about what is going to be done in the operating room in order to complete this part of your therapy.

The removal of the bladder and reconstruction of the urinary tract usually takes three to five hours. Although operations take more or less time depending upon the patient's physical characteristics, most experienced surgical teams complete the surgery in about this amount of time. You and your family should remember, however, that the preparation prior to the beginning of surgery usually takes about thirty minutes. Additional time is required after the operation to apply a sterile bandage to the incision site, awaken the patient from anesthesia, and then transport the patient to the recovery room. Consequently, the entire process from beginning to end could take anywhere from four to seven hours. After the patient arrives in the recovery room, further time is required to ensure that he or she is stable.

For family members waiting in the visitors room for a loved one undergoing surgery, the wait can be a long one. Our nurses and operating room staff attempt to keep family members up-to-date by calling out to the waiting rooms or actually visiting with patients' families during the procedure. You might ask your surgeon about such practices at the hospital where you plan to have surgery. Communication during the procedure can be reassuring to all involved.

Once the operation is over, patients generally spend twenty-four hours in the intensive care unit for postoperative monitoring. Not every hospital or surgeon recommends obligatory intensive care unit attention after cystectomy; this is a matter of hospital and physician preference and is determined largely by the patient's overall clinical condition and the outcome of the surgical procedure. Obviously, if unanticipated complications like significant bleeding or other problems occur during the operation, most urologists recommend intensive care unit monitoring for a period of time after surgery. Once the immediate postoperative period is over, the patient is usually transferred to a regular room for the remainder of the in-hospital recuperation. During this time, careful monitoring by physician, nursing staff, and members of the enterostomal therapy team (see chapter 6) will help the patient get ready for discharge from the hospital.

During the operation, a tube is passed into your nose and down into your stomach to drain the contents of your intestinal tract so that you do not develop postoperative bloating, nausea, and vomiting. This tube, called a *nasogastric tube*, usually remains in place for the first few days after surgery. It does not decrease the likelihood of developing a small bowel obstruction, but it has been shown in a number of studies to decrease the risk of postoperative discomfort associated with the bloating that results from the intestinal tract having been handled during surgery. The intestines, after having been manipulated during the operation, usually "go to sleep" for a period of time. Gradually, during the first few days after your operation, the intestines will "awaken" on their own and begin functioning again.

You will also notice other drains, placed at the time of surgery, coming out of your abdominal wall adjacent to the incision. These small tubes are usually connected to vacuum reservoirs made of plastic and serve to evacuate blood clots and serum that accumulate in the region of your operation immediately after surgery.

Depending upon the type of urinary tract reconstruction you have had, other drains may also be used to speed healing. For patients who choose a continent catheterizable reconstruction, a small catheter exiting the catheterization mechanism is used to keep this area open. Another larger tube, referred to as a *supra pubic catheter,* will exit through the new reservoir and the abdominal wall. Both of these tubes will be connected to drainage bags, and urine will collect in them continuously. If your surgeon has built a neobladder connected to your urethra, you'll have a catheter passing through the urethra into the neobladder. You will also have a suprapubic catheter similar to the one used for people with continent catheterizable reconstructions. In either case, the suprapubic catheter is used as a safety valve, to guarantee safe exit of urine from the bladder as healing occurs and to provide a method for easily measuring residual urine volumes after the urethral catheter has been removed and the patient begins to learn how to urinate again or how to evacuate the bladder by intermittent catheterization.

During your hospital stay, you will be taught to take care of your drains and, particularly if you had a complex reconstruction, you will need to learn how to care for or participate in the care of these tubes, as they will remain in place for a few weeks after you are discharged from the hospital. Most medical centers leave tubes in continent catheterizable reservoirs and in neobladders for two to three weeks following surgery. Because mucus from the intestinal tract can accumulate in reservoirs constructed from small or large intestines and block drainage catheters, your nurses and doctors will teach you how to efficiently flush sterile fluid through the tubes to ensure that obstructing mucus does not accumulate in your new bladder. It is important to understand that you will be responsible for flushing the reservoir when you go home, even if a home health aid or visiting nurse is scheduled to see you on a regular basis.

Over a period of about six to ten days, you will be asked to get out of bed and walk in the hall on a regular basis, and you will perform leg exercises to diminish the likelihood of developing a blood clot in your legs and breathing exercises to minimize the risk of developing postoperative pneumonia. You are given a diet of clear liquids in the beginning, but this is slowly advanced to a menu that approximates what you eat at home. Once normal intestinal function has returned and you have fully recovered, you are discharged. You should return about three weeks after surgery for a postoperative visit. After that, additional arrangements are made depending upon the type of reconstruction performed. Usually within four weeks of surgery, bladder drains and catheters are removed, and about six weeks after surgery you are able to turn to normal daily activities.

Follow-up

After the initial six-week recovery period, patients are usually asked to return every three to six months for five years so postoperative x-rays and laboratory studies can be done to determine their cancer has not returned and no significant metabolic abnormalities have resulted from their reconstruction. Follow-up after major bladder cancer surgery is usually a lifelong affair. After about five years, if the patient has shown no evidence of recurrent disease, the odds are good that the cancer will not return. Nonetheless, late recurrences are not unheard of. Consequently, patients who have had a cystectomy and a form of urinary tract reconstruction, whether it be an ileal conduit or a neobladder, need to stay in touch with their urologist.

CHAPTER SIX

Life after Urinary Tract Reconstruction

If you have had the bladder surgery described in chapter 5, you already know that you need to make some adjustments in your life and that some of them may be difficult or unpleasant. You may be afraid that things will never be "normal" for you again. In reality, though, "normal" is and always has been a moving target—we all have to make adjustments for various circumstances as we move through life.

How you adapt depends on your unique combination of physical, emotional, intellectual, and spiritual past experiences and present strengths and your support network of family and friends. It may help to remember you are not alone with your problems—almost 1 million people in North America are living with ostomies of some sort, and 70,000 new procedures are done each year. Many people find that the best way to control life-changing events such as a cystectomy is to become as well informed as possible about all aspects of the procedure and what will follow. Again, that is the primary reason we wrote this book.

At the end of this chapter we talk about how this surgery changes the lives of the people closest to the person who has had ostomy surgery. They too will have to make adjustments and think about how their life may be different now.

While this book addresses general concerns and the many issues related to ostomy and recovery that we have encountered in our medical practices, you may have specific questions that are not covered here. We suggest you make a list of these questions to take with you on your next visit with your physician or enterostomal therapy nurse. The enterostomal therapy (ET) nurse is part of a team that is specially trained to help you with your recovery and return to normal life.

Dealing with Stress

Life—with some adaptations—*will* return to normal after ostomy surgery. Although no one would say that the adjustment process is easy, being prepared does make it *easier*. As you get ready for this major step in your life, think about successful ways you have coped with stress in the past. Ask yourself a few questions:

—Does it help when you talk things out?
—Do you like a lot of information—or the minimum?
—To gather information, do you prefer to read on your own or ask questions of someone else?
—Is it helpful to talk with people who have been through the same thing?
—Are there special people in your family or community on whom you can rely?
—Do you tend to isolate yourself when stressed?
—Do you usually carry your burdens alone?
—Have you found counselors to be helpful in dealing with problems?
—What things do you most want from your doctor or other caregivers?

These are just some ideas about how different people handle stress, to get you thinking about what your own needs are and how to meet them. This is the time to begin to explore how you cope. And if you share this information with the people involved with your care, they will be able to provide support in the way that is most helpful to you.

With so many things happening to you, it may be hard to know where to focus. You are faced with a diagnosis of cancer and possible changes in your lifestyle. It may be difficult to think about the surgery and about life afterward when you are worried about what will be found in surgery and what those findings will mean to you. Although it is not realistic to think that you can set all of your concerns aside, you may very well feel less overwhelmed if you address them one by one. Which ones can be solved with someone else's help or by getting additional information? If you are afraid of pain, for example, you can talk with your doctor and let him or her know that you would like special care taken to make sure you have as little pain as possible. You may find that taking steps to alleviate even one of your concerns will provide relief and give you more emotional energy to cope with some other issues.

Although many couples say their battle with cancer brought them closer together and they gained a true appreciation for each other, there is no question that this experience puts tremendous stresses on a relationship. Ideally, if there are stresses already present, such as unfinished business or things you need to discuss with each other, you and your partner should resolve them before treatment begins. Problems cannot be solved overnight, but so often they seem to grow larger and more insurmountable when they are avoided. As one patient stated so eloquently, "The time to discuss jobs, position in the boat, and overall strategy is before you get to the white water."

Many people find it helpful to talk with others who have actually experienced the operation. The United Ostomy Association provides visitors for this purpose. Every attempt is made to match the visitor to the new patient as closely as possible. You may request a visitor and spouse to meet with you and your partner. Your local branch of the American Cancer Society will have information about support group meetings in your area.

Your Choices

If you know that you need your bladder removed but are not sure which operation is best, you may need to gather more information from the sources you feel most comfortable with. These are the factors considered in the choice of operation, which you may need to learn more about before you make a decision:

—the extent and location of your tumor in the bladder

—your lifestyle and activity preferences

—your age and sex

—the need for further treatment

—your general health and ability to tolerate anesthesia.

As we saw in the previous chapter, when the bladder is removed, either a conduit must be made so the urine can exit the body or a substitute bladder must be constructed. *Urostomy* is the general term used for the surgical procedure in which urine is diverted from the body's urinary system. The most common urostomy procedure is the external appliance ostomy, in which a conduit is made leading out of the body to an external pouch that catches the urine. This operation has been performed since the early 1950s, and for years it was the only option available to cystectomy patients. There are many names given to the external urostomy, and you may hear them all at various times: Bricker's pouch, ileal loop or conduit if a part of the ileum (small intestine) is used, and colonic loop or conduit if part of the colon (large intestine) is used. The majority of our bladder removals include external appliance ostomies; the patient's role in handling the appliance is discussed in detail in this chapter.

Today, with advances in technology and the development of new techniques, there are other options, including internal pouches. Internal pouches are usually constructed using a combination of colon (large intestine), or cecum, and ileum (small intestine). There are many names for and variations in the methods of performing these procedures, but they fall into two broad categories. One is the internal pouch with a stoma. With this procedure, the stoma must be catheterized at regular intervals to empty the pouch of urine. The other category is an internal pouch attached to the urethra. This option offers the prospect of continence through "voiding" at regular intervals by tensing abdominal muscles and passing urine through the urethra. A patient's suitability for internal pouches depends on the factors listed above.

If you have an internal pouch, your personal role in operating your urinary system will eventually return to close to what it was before the surgery. For the remainder of this chapter, then, we examine various aspects, technical and otherwise, involved in living with an external appliance ostomy.

External Appliance Ostomy

Choosing a Stoma Site

The stoma is the opening to the outside of the body through which the urine flows to the external collection device. The stoma, which is constructed from a piece of the bowel, as explained in the next section, is red and moist. Some people think it looks like pursed lips.

One of the most important things you will do before your operation is choose a stoma site. Your surgeon or ET nurse will examine your abdomen for scars, skin folds, belt line, and so on, and observe what changes occur in the contours as you sit, stand, and bend. A site is chosen in as smooth an area as possible, where movement will not interfere with the pouch seal. It is also important that you be able to see and reach the stoma well, so you can care for it.

The Urostomy Procedure

In chapter 5 we described what is done in a cystectomy. After the bladder has been removed, the second half of the procedure is spent constructing an alternative to get the urine out of the body. To begin, a piece of intestine must be separated from the intestinal tract in order to make the conduit. This separation is made with care to preserve the nerve and blood supply to this piece of bowel. The segment is closed at one end, and the other end is brought out through an opening in the abdomen that the surgeon has made on the spot preselected for the stoma.

Outside the body, the piece of bowel is turned back, in a way similar to folding a cuff, and stitched to the skin. This is the stoma. The conduit is also stitched at the other layers of tissue it passes through, making it very secure. Since the stoma is cuffed, the part you see is actually the inside lining of the bowel. This part of the bowel is strong and germ-resistant, as its original purpose was to pass along waste matter, so infection of the external bowel piece is not a concern.

The ureters are implanted into the back part of this piece of bowel so the urine can pass through. Amazingly enough, because the piece of bowel still has its nerve and blood supply, it still propels matter forward as it did when it was part of the intestinal tract. In this way, the piece of bowel helps keep the urine moving out of the body. This does not occur during the postsurgical period, however, because anesthesia temporarily stops all bowel activity for a few days. To facilitate healing of the ureter, during the operation the doctor usually places two long, thin plastic tubes through the connections between the ureters and the piece of intestine. These tubes can be seen coming out of the stoma, although they will be inside the plastic pouch and visible only when the pouch is changed. Often the doctor also places a shorter tube into the stoma to help drain any urine that may pool in the bowel segment. You won't feel the tubes, and most of the time they will be removed before you leave the hospital. Occasionally, if your doctor thinks you may not have healed enough, they will be left in a bit longer.

The ability of the bowel to propel the urine forward rather than allowing it to pool inside is vital in preventing urinary tract infection. In the coming years, your doctor will periodically order tests to assess whether this is happening as it should. This is one of the reasons people who have had this operation for bladder cancer need lifelong medical follow-up.

We described what takes place in a "bowel prep" for surgery in chapter 5. You can understand why this was necessary when you consider the need to remove as much bacteria as possible from your new conduit and from the area where your bowel has been joined back together. Having your intestines cleaned out prior to surgery also helps reduce the chance of other infection and severe gas pains.

After Ostomy Surgery

After your operation, you can expect a great deal of swelling in the pelvic area. For men, the rectum also may be affected because of its proximity to the prostate. The temporary swelling caused by the removal of the prostate sometimes affects sensation or tone in the rectum until the inflammation subsides and the rectal nerves recover.

We stated in chapter 5 that removal of the bladder and construction of the ileal conduit may take three to six hours. The length of time varies depending on your weight and whether you have had other abdominal operations, radiation, or injuries that may have caused internal adhesions or scarring. An ostomy pouch is attached to your abdomen before you leave the operating room, and the spout at the bottom is attached to tubing that leads to a collection bag hooked to the side of your bed. This makes it easier for your doctor and nurses to measure your urine output without disturbing you. They use this information to help determine if you are getting enough intraveneous fluid and if your kidneys are functioning well.

When you awaken from anesthesia, you will have many intravenous lines (IVs) going into your body. This is because of the large amount of IV fluid that you are given during the operation and the IV antibiotics you need to protect you from infection. You will also have a heart monitor attached for careful monitoring of your heart during the first twenty-four hours after surgery.

While you were under anesthesia, a breathing tube (endotracheal tube) was placed in your mouth to ensure that you get enough oxygen during the operation. This is usually removed as you are waking up, and most people do not remember it at all, although they may have a bit of a sore throat as a reminder that it was there. Also while you are under anesthesia, a smaller tube may have been passed through your nose into your stomach to keep your stomach empty. This tube may or may not be present when you wake up.

Learning Ostomy Care

After the operation, while you are still in the hospital, there are many things for you to learn. Your ET nurse will help guide the process, but you will be primarily responsible for the pace of your learning. There are many different emotional reactions to surgery. Some people feel that they need a day or two before they are ready to take on the tasks of life adjustment, while others can hardly wait to get started. In either case, the teaching and learning process will proceed in small steps tailored to meet your individual needs. If you are able to meet before surgery with the ET nurse who will be involved with your care and teaching afterward, you may wish to discuss with him or her your readiness and the ways you learn best.

The first bridge to cross in the adjustment process is looking at the stoma for the first time. By this time you will have seen a picture of a stoma or at least heard a description of one. You will remember that it is red and moist and that when you come out of surgery there are usually two or three small tubes protruding from it to help ensure a free flow of urine until healing takes place. Most people react to seeing the stoma by saying it's bigger than they thought it would be. Remember, the stoma is usually swollen at first and will shrink to its final size during the next four to six weeks. The time and amount of change varies from person to person. Your stoma may not change much at all, or it may eventually be only half its original size. When you touch the stoma, you will notice that you feel no sensation from it, even though it may look like it is sore and tender.

The pouch that was applied in the operating room is usually changed one or two days after surgery. This is your first opportunity to see the stoma.

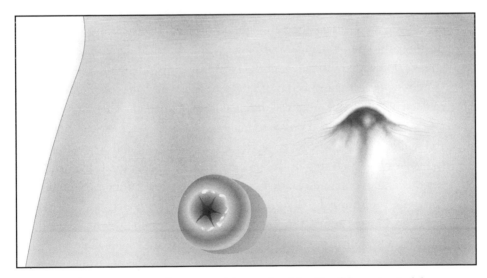

Fig. 6.1. A representation of a stoma exiting on the right side of the patient's abdomen, just below the patient's umbilicus (navel).

When the pouch is removed, the skin around the stoma (the *peristomal* area) is cleaned and prepared for the new pouch. This is done by simply washing the area with soap and water, rinsing it well, and drying it. It's a good idea to avoid highly perfumed or very creamy soaps, because they may cause itching or interfere with the pouch seal. People with extremely sensitive skin may choose to wash with water only. For these people, the the *peristomal* area may be coated with a liquid skin barrier or protector and allowed to dry.

The pouch is then prepared for application. The stoma is measured to be sure the pouch has the proper sized opening, and if necessary the pouch is cut to fit onto the stoma without allowing any skin to be exposed to urine. Sometimes a pectin-based wafer is also applied with the pouch for added skin protection. Precut pouches are available for those who do not want to bother cutting the opening each time. Some people cut the openings in their pouches while their stoma is changing size as swelling subsides and then switch to precut pouches a few weeks after surgery.

Very soon after surgery, perhaps the next day, you will be helped out of bed so you can walk around a bit. Even though you might feel weak and achy and would rather stay in bed, it is important to get up and walk around as soon as possible after surgery to help to keep your lungs clear. When you are feeling strong enough, you will probably want to stand up in the bathroom to change your pouch. This makes it easier to see what you are doing, and you may find the bathroom mirror helpful, too.

When you get out of bed or go for a walk in the hall, you might want to detach your pouch from the drainage tubing and bag. This is practical for two reasons: you won't have so much equipment to take with you, and you will gain more experience working with the spout and connector. In the beginning, each step in the process must be thought out. Eventually the process becomes automatic and takes only a few minutes. No one is born with the knowledge of how to change an ostomy pouch, and you may feel overwhelmed at first. Guided practice in the hospital will make it easier. We know from our years of clinical experience that you will be able to do it—just give yourself time and focus on mastering the necessary procedures one step at a time.

Going Home

For everyone who has had a urostomy with an external appliance, emptying the urine pouch becomes a continuing part of everyday life. Whether you are at home, at work, or at a party, you will need to empty your pouch every few hours. The timing is partially dependent on how much you've had to drink. Since it is always important to drink fluids—at least six to eight glasses of water a day are recommended unless your liquids are restricted for other reasons—you can count on needing to empty your pouch at least three to four times during the average day.

When you get home, you will have to make a decision about how you want to empty your pouch overnight. Many people choose to attach the pouch to drainage tubing and a bag or bottle while they are sleeping, so that the pouch stays empty. Your kidneys usually produce more urine during the night than the pouch can contain, so if you do not choose this option, you will have to get up at least once a night to empty. The choice in this matter is a personal one. One caution, however: Many people say they expect it will be easy to get up and empty the pouch because they are accustomed to awakening several times during the night anyway to go to the bathroom. It was likely the full, diseased bladder that had been awakening them, however, and they are surprised to find themselves sleeping through the night at home after surgery. If you don't use tubing, you may want to set an alarm.

> After a urostomy, it's a different thing in your life to get used to, but it's not a problem if you don't make it a problem. At first I was afraid to move around much. I was very afraid of activity because I was afraid it would leak. But you get the hang of it.

The pouches are made so that they are not noticeable through clothing, with hypoallergenic but strong adhesives that hold up through normal showering, bathing, exercise, or swimming. Virtually all disposable pouches manufactured today have antireflux valves or separate compartments that keep urine in the lower part of the pouch from getting back up to the stoma. Both clear and opaque pouches are available, and they come in a variety of shapes and textures and with a variety of adhesives. Two-piece pouches are also available, with the sticky portion and the collecting portion separated to allow one to change the size and shape of the pouch without removing the adhesive from the skin. Some people like to wear a larger clear pouch most of the time and switch to a smaller or opaque pouch during physical activity such as exercise or sexual intercourse.

Getting on with Life

There seems to be an unwritten but rigidly followed code when it comes to bodily eliminations. We learn very early in life that there is an expectation to be quiet, odor free, private, and—above all—in control. We pass through many phases in developing our personal code, from the jokes of elementary school to the stereotype of people becoming obsessed with elimination patterns as they grow older. We develop our personal beliefs and adjust them to fit cultural norms.

It is natural for anyone undergoing ostomy surgery to have concerns about how this will affect them in relationships and as a member of society. We have been taught to strive for the "body beautiful"—we want to be perfect "10s." In addition to fears about changes in appearance brought about by this surgery, the thought of possible loss of control and elimination taboos is a frightening one for most people.

Hearing about the pouch options available and learning self-care is the quickest way to regain the much-desired control. In the days following surgery and throughout your recuperation at home, as you become more and more competent at the tasks necessary for continuing ostomy care, your fears will decrease and you will begin to feel more in control of your bodily functions.

The type of pouch you wear is largely a personal preference, but if you have a partner or special person in your life the type of pouch you choose may be a joint decision. You may find that certain types feel better or meet your specific needs better than others. You want to choose a reliable, affordable, comfortable pouch. With encouragement, your partner will probably be frank with you about his or her own preferences about seeing the pouch and being involved in care. Although some people do not even want their spouses to see the pouch, others are much less self-conscious. Many attractive undergarments are available that cover the pouch during intimate moments. One former patient of ours told us of an incident when he was with a group of college friends who decided to "skinny dip." He recounted, "Before I knew it, I'd stripped down to my pouch and jumped in. No one seemed to notice!"

It is your decision to tell or not to tell. If you find the support of friends helpful, share your experiences, but no one need know if you choose not to discuss your surgery. There is no right or wrong way to handle this personal decision.

Pouches are emptied as needed during the course of a day and should be changed every three to four days. Wearing the pouch longer than that may lead to urinary tract infection owing to the bacteria that grows in the pouch over time. After you have become familiar with the process, changing your pouch will only take a few minutes. You may wish to combine the task with showering. Although you may develop a twice-a-week routine for changing your pouch, most people carry an emergency kit with them for unexpected situations. The more at ease you become with the changing procedure and your equipment, the less likely you will be to have leaks. However, we advise our patients to think preventively—just as you would take an umbrella on a picnic in case of rain, keep an extra pouch with you in case of leaks.

As you leave the hospital and begin your new life, it is normal to have many concerns and fears about the future and your ability to cope with it. Many people experience an emotional letdown after they get home. Activities like taking walks (malls are great for this in bad weather), going to your place of worship, or going out to dinner or the movies are important steps toward adjustment. You may feel you have to force yourself to get out and do something, but if you don't, you'll soon start to feel that you can't. Sometimes the only way to convince yourself that you are okay and that no one knows you have an ostomy bag is to get out with other people. You'll be amazed at how oblivious people can be to changes that seem major to you.

Exercise is an important part of recovery. Walking is good for the body as well as the spirit. It is the best early postoperative exercise. People are always surprised to find that although they have lost weight during their hospital stay, their waistlines have somehow mysteriously enlarged. Walking first, with the gradual addition of leg lifts in a few weeks, is a great way to regain tone in those stretched and traumatized abdominal muscles. Most preoperative activities may be resumed within a month of surgery. You may want to avoid weight lifting or activities that could result in a blow to the abdomen. One of our patients resumed karate lessons but took the precaution of wearing a hard athletic cup over his stoma.

You may feel very close to your doctor, ET nurse, and other caretakers after going through so much that is so personal with them. They help you relearn to eliminate. A female member of our team had spent many hours in the bathroom with one particular patient. One day he needed to empty his pouch and she accompanied him to the bathroom, as usual. She knew he was ready for graduation when he said, "Would you mind turning your back? I don't like to pee in front of a woman."

Diet

There are no dietary adjustments that will be necessary because you have had a urostomy. In the first weeks after your operation, however, you may want to avoid hard-to-digest foods or high-fiber foods. Small quantities may be all right, but test the effects before eating large amounts. Remember that you have had abdominal surgery and your body needs to readjust to the eating process.

Fluid intake is very important. The best way to prevent infections and kidney stone formation is to keep urine flowing through the system. After your bladder is gone you may be more prone to urinary tract infection. The urine of a person who takes in enough fluids is normally slightly acidic. This acidity prevents germs from flourishing in the urine. Unless your fluid intake is restricted for other reasons, make an effort to drink at least six to eight glasses of liquid a day. Many people who have had bladder problems have gotten into the bad habit of withholding liquids in order to decrease the number of trips to the bathroom. In fact, very few people drink as much as they should for optimum urinary tract health. When you have had a urostomy, however, it becomes even more important to drink! drink! drink!

So long as it is not alcohol, which dehydrates the body, the type of fluid is not critical unless you have had kidney stones in the past and your doctor has adjusted your diet to help prevent stone formation. Many people have heard that people with urostomies must drink cranberry juice. Although cranberry juice does seem to deodorize the urine, one would have to drink gallons of it before it would have an effect on the pH (acidity) of the urine. Certain foods—for example, asparagus—may affect the odor of urine. Some medications, particularly antibiotics, may change the color or odor of urine. If you notice odor or color changes, think first of what you have eaten or if you have started a new medication. Increase your fluid intake. Your urine may be darker or have an odor simply because you are not drinking adequate amounts. If the change persists for over twenty-four hours or if you cannot identify the cause, call your urologist.

Potential Problems Ahead

Patients are most likely to have one of the following three problems after they have been discharged from the hospital: blood in the urine, stoma irritations, or bowel problems. You need to be aware of these problems not because you *are likely* to have one or more of them but because you *may* have one of them. Since the possibility exists, you need to know what to look for and what to do.

Blood or Other Abnormalities in Urine

During the time in the hospital, your urine is bloody because of the surgery. By the time you leave the hospital or within a few days thereafter, your urine should be clear of blood. Though it may always appear a bit cloudy because of mucus produced by the piece of bowel used to form your urostomy, the following symptoms may be signs of an infection. You should call your doctor if:

—you notice blood in your urine not related to trauma to the stoma (for example, bumping it), or the amount of mucus increases a great deal

—you notice a foul smell to your urine
—you have a fever
—you have pain in the kidney area

Stoma Irritations

Occasionally, particularly as you are learning to manage pouch changes, you may develop skin or stoma irritations. If you are unable to remedy these using instructions given to you in the hospital, call your ET nurse for advice. The type and location of any irritated areas may give clues as to the cause and solution.

Bowel Problems

The most common complaints people have when they return for their first doctor visit after surgery have to do with bowel-related problems. Most people have diarrhea or constipation after surgery, owing to the swelling and stresses associated with the procedure. Usually these problems resolve within a few weeks after surgery, but some people who are constipated may have to take a gentle laxative. Although these problems are expected, they may have other causes; diarrhea may be due do antibiotics, or constipation may result from dehydration. Especially in the early weeks after surgery, check with your surgeon before treating yourself.

Follow-up

It is important to see your urologist and ET nurse at regular intervals after surgery. As the years pass the visits may become less frequent, but they are still necessary to maintain good urologic health and discover minor problems before they become large ones.

A Word to the Partner

You may feel during this process that you are going through all the same adjustments as your loved one who is having surgery. In fact, you are. You will certainly be riding the same emotional roller coaster and be worried about the same things. Do not underestimate or ignore your needs at this time. Though you are concerned for your partner, be sure to allow time for yourself—stop, have lunch with a friend, recharge your batteries.

Although many people try to do everything for the "sick" person, you may find this is not the best approach for your own or your partner's mental health. The key to rebuilding self-esteem for a patient is returning as quickly as possible to the pre-illness level of self-care and independence. Be aware of the many taboos related to elimination (from bowels or bladder) in our culture. Self-care of the ostomy is important as a way of feeling that things are returning to the usual or normal pattern. Sexual relationships are of concern to most people having ostomy surgery. As the partner, you can immediately begin to re-establish your loving relationship by discussing what involvement with the ostomy your partner wants you to have. This may be watching the first pouch change, if you are both comfortable with that, or shopping for a sexy undergarment for the partner, who might be fearful of your rejection.

It could be some time after surgery (depending on age, physical condition, and overall recovery) before you know if you will be able to resume the same kind of sexual activity you enjoyed before the operation. Cuddling, kissing, back rubs, and hand-holding are good ways to reinitiate closeness and are very satisfying to many people. Women who have had cystectomies may complain of painful intercourse the first few times it is attempted after surgery. One woman described it as the same way it had felt trying intercourse for the first time after having had a baby. Men may have some discomfort in the pelvis and may tire easily at first. Patience and plenty of rest are the keys. For patients of either sex, a gentle, supportive approach by the partner is helpful.

People are afraid of leaks from their pouch during sexual activity. Our response to this is a variance of an old line: there are actually three things you have to do in life—die, pay taxes, and empty your pouch before sex! For the person with an ostomy, spontaneous sex takes at least a little planning.

While there is no denying that urostomy is a life-changing procedure for anyone, it is also true that gradually, as you heal, you will be able to resume all of the activities of your life before surgery. Share any concerns or questions you have about your life after surgery with your partner, your doctor, or your nurse, and take advantage of other community resources if you feel they will help.

CHAPTER SEVEN

Bladder-Preserving Strategies

In an ideal world, surgeons would be able to remove tumors and malignant tissue without disturbing the organs that are important to healthy body functioning. In reality, as we have seen, this is often an impossible challenge. However, the quest continues, with some success: increasingly, new approaches that remove cancers but leave organs intact are being used successfully. In a search for organ-preserving approaches in the management of tumors, physicians have combined less aggressive surgical procedures with radiation and chemotherapy. Breast cancer, sarcomas of the limbs, and cancers of the anus are among the kinds of cancers being managed by this organ-preserving approach. Patients who previously would have been treated with radical surgical procedures like mastectomy or amputation of a limb are now treated with radiation after limited surgery. Some patients also receive chemotherapy.

In many cases, organ-preserving approaches have proved just as effective as more extensive surgery and have preserved function and body image to a great extent. The same principles are now being applied to the treatment of bladder cancer. We now often hold off more radical surgical procedures such as the cystectomy, keeping it as an alternative for patients whose tumors do not respond to organ-preserving therapy or for patients whose tumors recur after the therapy. A cystectomy after treatment with organ-preserving therapy is called *salvage therapy*.

Background

Historically, the nonsurgical treatment for muscle-invasive bladder cancer has been radiation therapy. Radiation therapy alone has been shown to effectively shrink bladder tumors. Survival rates for patients treated with either radiation alone or surgery alone are about the same, but a large number of patients treated only with radiation require surgery later because of local tumor recurrence. Therefore, while most bladder tumors have a good response when treated with radiation alone and some patients are actually cured, the greater likelihood of local tumor recurrence makes the use of radiation alone a less than perfect approach in preventing tumor recurrence locally in the pelvis.

Chemotherapy after a tumor biopsy has also been used in the treatment of bladder cancer in an attempt to avoid either radical surgery or radiation. While there has been some limited success with this approach, frequently tumors recur in the bladder, making it necessary for the patient to have either bladder removal surgery or radiation.

In recent years, studies have investigated a combination approach in the treatment of patients with muscle-invasive bladder cancer. These studies take a three-pronged approach:

—local resection of the tumor (transurethral resection, or TUR, as explained in chapter 4)
—radiation
—chemotherapy

Radiation and chemotherapy used together as a bladder-preserving technique are proving to be much more effective than either radiation or chemotherapy alone. The balance of this chapter focuses on this combination, known as the *chemoradiation approach.*

The primary goal of any cancer treatment is to cure the patient of his or her tumor. An organ-preserving technique should only be undertaken when the likelihood of cure using this method is equivalent to the likelihood of cure using a more radical approach. It is also important to preserve the quality of bladder function throughout the therapy. It would be of little value if the patient were cured of bladder cancer by bladder-preservation techniques but ended treatment with a nonfunctioning bladder, requiring removal of that bladder later.

Predicting Success: Who Can Benefit

Some tumors can be more successfully treated than other tumors with bladder-sparing therapies using combination chemotherapy and radiation. One of the most important indicators for success is the completeness of the transurethral resection of the tumor. In studies, it appears that patients who had received a complete, or total, resection of the tumor at the time of cystoscopy have the best results. This makes sense because the better or more complete the resection, the fewer malignant cells left behind for the radiation and chemotherapy to treat.

Tumor location is another factor that appears to be related to outcome. In part, this is linked to the first factor. For example, tumors located at or near the ureteral orifice cause ureteral obstruction and *hydronephrosis*, a back-up of fluid into the kidneys causing the kidneys to become distended. Patients with tumors in this location do not seem to do as well with bladder-preservation therapy. This may be due to doctors' inability to completely excise tumors in this location by TUR without causing irreparable bladder harm. Therefore, it is generally recommended that patients with hydronephrosis caused by tumor obstruction undergo radical cystectomy rather than bladder preservation.

The stage of the tumor also seems to be a factor. Patients whose tumors are in the T_2 and early T_3 category tend to fare better with the combination bladder-sparing approach than patients whose tumors are in the T_4 category. Again, this is likely because a more complete TUR can be performed in patients with early-stage tumors, decreasing the number of tumor cells remaining to be killed by chemoradiation.

Finally, patients whose tumors begin to shrink after an initial course of chemotherapy and radiation are thought to have a better outcome after bladder-conserving treatment than those whose tumors have minimal or no response. While some tumors take longer to respond than others, it makes practical sense to continue to treat patients whose tumors show a good response to therapy.

The First Steps in Bladder-Preservation Therapy

To decide if you are a candidate for bladder-preservation therapy, your urologist will conduct a thorough evaluation. The first few steps in any evaluation include procedures you have by now become familiar with as you have moved through the medical system: a complete history and a physical examination, which will focus on the signs and symptoms of bladder cancer and any indications about the extent of the tumor's spread. Standard blood work should be performed, including kidney function analysis and complete blood counts. A chest x-ray and CT scan or MRI scan of the pelvis should be performed to assess the extent of tumor spread.

Once these studies have been evaluated, a urologic surgeon familiar with bladder cancer management performs a cystoscopic evaluation of the bladder. This is the critical first step in a bladder-preservation program. The urologist identifies and maps the location of the tumor for future reference, to allow for more accurate examinations and biopsy to aid in planning for radiation. A transurethral resection (TUR) of the tumor is then performed as completely as possible. As noted earlier, a successful outcome depends heavily on the completeness of this TUR. Next, a pathologic evaluation of the tumor specimen is performed, and the extent of tumor spread is noted. Bladder muscle invasion and the depth of that invasion are two critical components of the pathologic review. Each of these factors affects the likelihood of successful treatment.

Making decisions about chemotherapy will be the next step in determining the course of bladder-preservation treatment. The use of chemotherapy in the bladder-preserving approach of combination chemoradiation serves several purposes. To varying degrees, chemotherapy itself can shrink bladder tumors. The use of two or more types of chemotherapeutic drugs together (known as *combination chemotherapy* or *multidrug regimens*) has been found to be more effective than using a single chemotherapy drug alone. It is also hoped that the chemotherapy, since it treats the whole body, will attack and wipe out any metastatic cells that may have escaped the bladder. An additional role that chemotherapy plays is to serve as a *radiosensitizer*—it helps the radiation work better by sensitizing the cells to some of the effects of radiation.

There are several types of chemotherapy used in these multidrug regimens. The most common chemotherapeutic drug in use for the treatment of bladder cancer is cisplatinum. This drug is often combined with two other drugs, methotrexate and vinblastine, in what is called the CMV regimen. In chapter 8, on chemotherapy, we will provide more details about how chemotherapy is administered and what the side effects can be.

Radiation's role in bladder cancer therapy is to kill the bladder cancer cells both inside the bladder and outside, in the tissue around the bladder. Local lymph nodes are also frequently treated as part of the therapy, to help address any microscopic cancer cells that may reside in them.

How Radiation Works

The type of radiation used to treat bladder cancer is actually x-rays, just like those used for imaging bones or obtaining a chest x-ray. However, the x-rays used for radiation treatment purposes are special high-energy x-rays, which are much more powerful and penetrating than those used for imaging. X-rays used to treat bladder cancer should be at an energy of six megavolts (six million volts) or greater. There are usually fewer skin reactions with this very high-energy, deeply penetrating radiation than were seen many years ago with lower-energy x-rays and cobalt machines.

One way that the high-energy radiation kills cancer cells is by damaging the cells' DNA. The DNA, as explained in chapter 2, is the part of the cell required for cellular life and reproduction; if the DNA is damaged, the cell can no longer perform these functions. Damaged DNA can also send signals to the cell to kill itself, a kind of cellular suicide. This might sound violent and painful, but radiation therapy is painless, even while cancer cells are being killed by the radiation. Receiving radiation therapy feels similar to a chest x-ray—that is, you won't feel a thing. However, after radiation you may experience side effects; these are explained later in this chapter.

The first step in preparing for radiation therapy is the planning session, or simulation. At this session, the radiation oncologist gathers information to decide what area to treat and how the treatment will be delivered. The simulation is carried out on the simulator machine, which is exactly like the machine that will be used for treatment, except that instead of delivering high-energy radiation it takes regular x-rays in order to identify anatomy.

Several procedures are generally performed at the time of simulation, to identify the bladder and surrounding structures more fully: First, the patient drinks an oral contrast material similar to barium in order to identify the location of the small intestine and make accommodations so that it can be shielded from treatment. Then contrast material is injected into the rectum, likewise to identify its location precisely so it can be shielded as much as possible. Finally, a catheter is placed into the bladder and the bladder is filled with a special waterlike contrast agent and with air so that the precise outlines of the bladder can be identified.

Once these organ localization techniques are complete, a leg and pelvis immobilization device is fashioned. This is used to minimize the patient's movement during treatment and to make it easier to position the patient in exactly the same spot for treatment each day. This immobilization device can be one of several types, including a plasticlike material that fully encases the pelvis and legs or a Styrofoam-like material that is formed around the contours of the pelvis and legs.

After the anatomic localization and immobilization processes are complete, the radiation oncologist decides how and where to treat. He or she designs a field—the area to be treated—and takes several special types of x-rays for continued planning and to record where and what is to be treated. Once the physician is satisfied with the location of the sites, special temporary marks are made on the patient's skin with an ink marker, identifying the treatment area. Several small permanent tattoo dots are also applied to the areas of the field. These tattoo dots are about the size of the dot on the letter *i* on this page and assist in positioning the patient appropriately each day.

The simulation process usually takes about one hour to complete. When it is over, the patient goes home and a team comprising the radiation oncologist, a physicist, and a *dosimetrist* (treatment planner) uses sophisticated computer programs to determine which organs will receive what dose of radiation, how many fields will be used, and at what angles the radiation will be delivered during the treatment. The computer programs also help determine which areas will be shielded from receiving radiation, which energy of radiation will be used, what amount of radiation will be delivered per day, and what will be the final dose of radiation.

The shielding (blocking) is designed to prevent or limit radiation exposure of certain organs while maintaining full radiation dose to the bladder and any other areas requiring treatment. There are two ways to provide the required shielding. One is the custom fabrication of lead alloy blocks cut to correspond exactly to areas of the individual patient's anatomy. A more recently developed shielding method is something called *multileaf collimation*. This type of shielding system employs fifty-two independently moving "fingers" of metal alloy that are housed in the head of the treatment machine (which is called a *linear accelerator*) and can be moved to match any blocking scheme. The advantage of this type of shielding is that the radiation therapist running the machine is not required to put blocks in the machine and later remove them for each field on each patient, as with multileaf collimation this is done automatically in the head of the machine. This decreases the overall treatment time for the patient, allowing for improved patient comfort and more accurate treatment.

The time between simulation and the first day of treatment can vary, but it is usually about three to five days. This allows enough time for the computer planning and shielding to be completed. During your radiation therapy, you will receive treatment every day but not necessarily exactly the same treatment every day. There are several procedures that occur daily and some that occur less frequently (once or twice per week).

In the first step of treatment, the patient undresses from the waist down and is positioned. The marks and tattoos on the skin, along with the immobilization device, allow for accurate and reproducible daily setup and positioning. Laser lights are used to help guide the positioning to within a very few millimeters of accurate repositioning each day. Once the patient is positioned, specialized x-rays called *port films* are done to again verify positioning at the desired location (determined from the simulation process) and to make any adjustments as necessary. When positioning is correct, actual treatment begins.

The linear accelerator makes a number of noises while operating. Parts of the machine, including the head, or gantry, and the table, also may move during the treatment.

The radiation therapist describes all these noises and movements before treatment begins. The treatment is delivered through several different fields, or angles, in order to concentrate the dose around the target without giving too much radiation to other organs or tissue in the body. In general, patients with bladder cancer are treated with three or four fields, usually one from the front, one from the back, and one from each side. The total time that the radiation beam is on to deliver the treatment is about six minutes. The total time that the patient spends on the table for positioning and treatment is about ten to twelve minutes.

While undergoing radiation treatment, patients are examined by the radiation oncologist once a week to assess any side effects of treatment or new symptoms. Suggestions for management of any side effects will be offered, including alterations in diet or medications that may help alleviate symptoms. Typically, however, few, if any, medications are required. Often, decreasing the amount of fiber in the diet, such as that found in fresh fruits and vegetables, can help minimize any loose stool or diarrhea.

Course of Treatment

A typical treatment course of chemoradiation for bladder preservation proceeds in the following steps, although exact timing and doses vary for different patients.

1. After the appropriate staging and workup has been completed and you have chosen to undergo a bladder-preserving approach as definitive therapy for your bladder cancer, the next step is to begin chemotherapy. As we explained, the most effective regimens have been found to be those that use more than one drug. Cisplatinum is usually one of the drugs. You receive the multidrug chemotherapy for several days and then receive no chemotherapy for about three weeks.

2. After the three-week break, the chemotherapy cycle is then repeated.

3. After the second cycle of multidrug chemotherapy, you begin the combination chemoradiation therapy. The standard course of radiation includes treatments five days per week along with cisplatinum

or cisplatinum and one other drug. During this time, the radiation is treating the entire bladder, perivesicular area, and local pelvic lymph nodes.

4. After about four to five weeks of chemoradiation, your doctor will examine and test you to evaluate the response of the tumor to this therapy. This evaluation includes a cystoscopy and biopsy, often a pelvic CT or MRI scan, and a chest x-ray. If there is no evidence of tumor, you will continue with the treatment for about two to three more weeks. However, if the tumor remains and there is little or no evidence of response to treatment, then a cystectomy is usually recommended at that time. This "salvage" cystectomy would be performed because it makes little sense to continue the chemoradiation when there is no evidence that the tumor is responding.

The side effects of the radiation can be separated into two groups: acute side effects, which occur during treatment, and late side effects, which occur months or years after treatment. Every individual responds differently to chemotherapy and radiation, and the side effects you will experience cannot be predicted. The more common possible side effects are listed in Table 7.1. Rarely will any one patient experience all the side effects noted.

It is important to realize that even with this attempt to spare the bladder, if the tumor does not respond to this therapy a cystectomy will be necessary. Fortunately, several studies have shown no evidence that delaying a cystectomy in the attempt to avoid radical surgery is harmful or decreases survival.

Yet the results with this type of chemoradiation for a bladder-preserving approach are encouraging. The overall survival of patients treated this way is about the same as it is in patients who undergo a cystectomy. About 75 percent of the patients who are able to complete the total combined chemoradiation therapy have no further evidence of invasive cancer and retain bladder function.

Patients whose tumors completely disappear after the initial portion of the treatment (chemotherapy and four to five weeks of radiation) are those who are most likely to successfully complete the entire course of therapy, remain cancer-free, and maintain a well-functioning bladder. It is rare that

Table 7.1 Possible Side Effects of Chemoradiation
for Bladder Cancer

Side effects during treatment	% Risk
Related to Radiation	
Bladder irritation	30
Diarrhea	25
Fatigue	20
Decreased white blood cell count	10
Blood in urine	10
Related to Chemotherapy	
Nausea	75
Decreased white blood cell count	35
Oral ulcers	25
Diarrhea	10
Side effects that can be long term (months or years)	
Impotence (depends on age and pretreatment potency status)	20–50
Occasional rectal bleeding	2–5
Poorly functioning bladder	2
Vaginal dryness	rare
Small intestine damage	rare

following chemoradiation a patient will require a cystectomy because of poor bladder function. The most common reason for a cystectomy after chemoradiation is recurrent, invasive bladder cancer. Superficial tumors may occur after bladder-sparing therapy but can almost always be managed by a cystoscopy, a transurethral resection (TUR), and intravesical therapy.

Life after Treatment

The treatments might be over, but not the regular and frequent visits to the doctors. Once bladder-preserving therapy has been completed, patients are advised to adhere to a fairly strict regimen of regular examinations and cystoscopic evaluations. For the first two years after treatment, these examinations are usually scheduled about every three months. A CT or an MRI scan of the abdomen and pelvis and chest x-ray are performed three months after ending treatment, and then again every six months.

This close follow-up continues for two years, and doctor visits are then extended to every six months until five years posttreatment, and then once per year. This intensity of follow-up is required to detect any new tumor growth that may require treatment or cystectomy.

Combined chemoradiation after TUR is a promising course of treatment with a substantial and growing amount of evidence to support its use in selected patients. Ideal patients are those with stage T_2 or T_3a cancers that do not obstruct the ureter. As we use this therapy on more and more patients, it is likewise becoming clear that certain patients may not be ideal candidates for this approach. These include patients with hydronephrosis and advanced (T_4) tumors.

Radical cystectomy remains the standard therapy for muscle-invasive bladder cancer in the United States, against which all other forms of treatment are judged. Combination chemoradiation remains a viable but less studied approach. Three-dimensional conformal radiation therapy and new, more highly active chemotherapeutic agents are becoming increasingly available and are undergoing study. These advances will continue to make the option of bladder-preserving therapy more attractive and possible.

CHAPTER EIGHT

Principles of Chemotherapy

The diagnosis of cancer can be a very frightening experience. If you learn that you or a loved one has cancer, many thoughts may run through your mind. Often these are misconceptions, gleaned from television or movie versions of cancer and cancer treatment. We find two common—and often erroneous—ideas that people have about cancer: that they will inevitably die from it and that the treatment can be worse than the disease.

Our objective here is to talk candidly about chemotherapy for bladder cancer, to dispel some myths while providing realistic and honest information. We begin with the true statement that the future has never looked brighter for people with cancer. Increasing numbers of new agents with significant power to fight bladder cancer are emerging, as are new ways to support patients and alleviate side effects through their treatments.

Who Will Treat You?

As noted in the introduction to this book, patients with cancer are cared for and treated by three groups of physicians: the urologist / surgeon, the radiation oncologist, and the medical oncologist. Let's look at medical treatment again in the context of chemotherapy. For many patients, the urologist or surgeon is the central physician guiding the care. The urologist usually performs the cystoscopy and biopsy to make the diagnosis and then, based on pathology reports, fully stages the disease, identifying the extent of its spread. If the tumor has remained localized to the superficial layers of the bladder, a patient is unlikely to require the assistance of the radiation oncologist or medical oncologist.

If superficial disease does not respond to surgery alone, the urologist may use chemotherapy, instilling the agents into the bladder and thereby exposing only the bladder lining to the drugs. A medical oncologist is not really needed for this type of chemotherapy administration. (This procedure is explained in chapter 4.) If the tumor extends through the wall or muscle of the bladder, however, the urologist collaborates closely with the radiation oncologist and the medical oncologist.

The role of the radiation oncologist is similar to the role of the surgeon, in that he or she works to control local symptoms related to the disease. (Radiation therapy for the urinary bladder is fully discussed in chapter 7.) Radiation is often given in combination with either surgery or chemotherapy. Patients with advanced disease that has spread outside the bladder to distant sites such as bone also may receive radiation therapy to those areas if symptoms occur. In these cases, radiation also prevents symptoms such as fractures of the bone from tumor growth.

The primary responsibilities of the medical oncologist in treating locally advanced and metastatic bladder cancer are: to determine the most appropriate chemotherapy regimen; to administer chemotherapy; and then to monitor the patient for side effects or adverse reactions. Surgery and radiation are *local* therapies, attacking the cancer at *specific sites*. Chemotherapy differs in that it is a *systemic* approach to attacking cancer cells, *involving the whole body*. It is usually given by mouth, through a vein, or under the skin, in order to use the bloodstream to deliver the cancer-attacking drugs to tumor sites. Systemic chemotherapy has the goal of seeking out the cancer cells wherever they may be.

In many cases, the places in the body where cancer has spread have been identified using scans, and these are the targets of therapy. Chemotherapy can also attack unknown sites of disease, microscopic deposits of cancer cells which are too small for the scanning methods to detect. Chemotherapy drugs affect, or kill, cancer cells at a higher rate than they do normal cells. For the most part, normal cells recover after chemotherapy. Cancer cells do not; if the drug is effective, they are permanently damaged. This balance of ridding the body of cancer and keeping the patient well usually can be maintained if the principles of chemotherapy are followed closely.

Medical oncologists sometimes feel they have gotten a bad rap over the years. It's the old blame-the-messenger syndrome. While new drugs and techniques have developed over the years and many medications have proven effective in diminishing or alleviating side effects, the fact remains that there are unpleasant aspects of chemotherapy for nearly everyone. Another fact is that, in exchange for this unpleasantness, no one can guarantee the results. The drugs you will be given have been prescribed because evidence shows they can be effective in combating cancer. But each cancer is an individual and sometimes very stubborn disease that doesn't always follow what we think should be the rules. Some people think of the oncologist as the person who makes them weak, miserable, and hairless, and then still cannot prevent them from dying. But many patients also bond with their oncologists, feeling—correctly—that this is the person who can be their most important ally in their fight against cancer.

Why Chemotherapy?

Chemotherapy makes a lot of sense in the treatment of bladder cancer. Bladder cancer is categorized as a disease that is moderately chemosensitive. Many drugs, alone or in combination with others, have a known ability to reduce tumor size, induce remission, and possibly cure patients of their disease. Newer agents that are undergoing early clinical testing appear promising, particularly in decreasing side effects while improving effectiveness against cancer cells. Because of these successes, chemotherapy is also offered in combination with surgery, radiation, or both (see chapter 7). Chemotherapy may make radiation more effective. As you read the rest of this chapter, the positive role chemotherapy plays in treating bladder cancer will become clear, along with the importance of the medical oncologist in the cancer care team.

The medical oncologist evaluates many factors before offering and initiating chemotherapy. Just because someone has cancer and there are drugs available to treat the cancer, it does not mean that chemotherapy will or should be offered. The tendency for toxicity and differing probabilities of response make the decision to embark on chemotherapy an individualized and personal one. Patients need to understand what the goals of therapy are, which side effects are likely to occur, and what alternatives are available. We encourage patients to ask questions.

Your physician should provide you the opportunity to discuss goals, options, and side effects of therapy. You should meet the staff who will be taking care of you in the clinic and, if necessary, the staff in the hospital. A reasonable team of caregivers would include your oncologist, an oncological nurse, a nutritionist, a pharmacist, and, should you require one, a social worker to assist with nonmedical but medically associated issues such as finances and insurance, support networks, and counseling. Physical therapists can be useful in providing information and support to maintain strength and maximize your potential during and after therapy.

Definition of Treatment Terms

To assist in your discussions with your health care team, the following terms and definitions concerning chemotherapy and other treatments may be useful:

—*Adjuvant therapy* is therapy offered to patients with a high risk for relapse after complete removal of all signs of the tumor, usually through surgery. Chemotherapy in the months following removal of the tumor has been found to help prevent or delay tumor recurrence for many types of cancer. It has been hard to prove this point in patients with bladder cancer, but this therapy has helped many colon and breast cancer patients, so it is also used for some bladder cancer patients.

Adjuvant therapy can sometimes be tough on the patient. After all, someone might be cancer-free and not need this extra therapy. They may feel they are suffering side effects for nothing. Or they may go through all the side effects and still have their disease come back. The decision about adjuvant therapy is based on odds and risks for improvement, balanced by how bad the side effects of therapy are.

Adjuvant therapy may also be frustrating because, since all signs of the tumor are gone, we really can't tell if it is working. With advanced or visible disease, we can look at radiographic scans and evaluate response.

—*Clinical trials* have three phases. Phase 1 trials are designed to find the safest dose of a drug to give patients. Often the dose is escalated throughout the trial, so people entering the trial early may have fewer side effects and possibly fewer responses, while patients entering late in a trial may receive a higher dose and have many side effects. Side effects and tumor response are not necessarily correlated. While it may seem logical that a higher dose of any drug is better, we do not know if this is true for many new drugs.

Once a drug has been found safe and the schedule for administering the drug has been determined, the drug enters phase 2 clinical trials. These trials test how often the drug at that dose and on that schedule causes tumors to shrink or improves symptoms. This is how response rates are determined. When the doctor tells you that drug x and y work 40 percent of the time, that data probably came from a phase 2 study.

If a drug looks effective in phase 2, it moves to phase 3, in which it is compared to the current therapy for the disease, to determine which regimen is best at shrinking tumors and improving survival. For patients considering participating in clinical trials, phase 3 studies should be offered first, then phase 2 if available, and finally phase 1 therapies. You should be told if you are receiving experimental therapies. In fact, if you are part of a research study, you will be asked to give formal consent after reading an explanation of the procedure for therapy, the risks, the benefits, and the alternatives. Typically there are more phase 1 studies than phase 2 or 3 studies.

—*Complete response* is defined as shrinkage of all measurable disease, that is, all visible evidence of the tumor is gone. This is similar to the term *remission* used in patients with leukemia. A complete response does not equal a cure, but you will not be cured unless there is a complete response. Patients who remain free of disease five years past diagnosis are considered cured. This "cure" is no guarantee, but only a very small percentage of people will ever have a recurrence of their disease past this time.

—*Cure* means being free of tumor—by whatever means—without recurrence for at least five years.

—*Cycle* is defined as a full course of therapy that is often repeated. Cycles are usually identified by days, either a twenty-one-day or twenty-eight-day cycle. It is during that cycle that treatment is given, side effects are observed and treated, and the patient recovers and gets ready for the next cycle. A cycle may vary in terms of the treatment schedules it contains. For example, the most commonly used regimen in advanced bladder cancer consists of four drugs, with one drug given on day one of the cycle, three other drugs given on day two, and two of those drugs given on days fifteen and twenty-two of the twenty-eight-day cycle. A different regimen may start with chemotherapy given on days one or two of the cycle and repeated every twenty-one days. Often, two cycles are given and then the state of response is evaluated prior to the third cycle of therapy.

—*Experimental therapy* is offered in the context of a clinical trial if standard therapy does not work. You may receive other therapy that your doctor has little experience with, but this is not considered experimental therapy; rather, new or experimental therapies are treatments that have shown promise in research laboratories against cancer cells living in test tubes or in animals and are now ready to be tested to see if they shrink tumors in humans.

—*Hospice* is a type of care focused on medical and social concerns at the end of life. It is begun when there is an understanding that real options for the treatment of the cancer are unlikely to work and that good care and relief of the symptoms of the patient need to be attended to.

—*Neoadjuvant therapy* is therapy offered before removal of the tumor. In this case, therapy may be used to make the tumor smaller and possibly easier to remove completely at the time of surgery. Neoadjuvant therapy also provides information on how chemosensitive a tumor is to therapy. In some cases, the chemotherapy works well enough to induce a complete remission and avoid surgery. However, the goal of neoadjuvant therapy is not organ preservation but tumor eradication using an approach that combines surgery and chemo. So far neoadjuvant therapy has not been found to play a significant role for patients with advanced bladder cancer.

—*Palliative care* refers to the services and treatment provided to patients to manage their symptoms and improve quality of life when cure is not likely. Patients with cancer do not have to suffer. They can have their symptoms managed and palliated. Palliative care is active therapy with the patient in mind. Sometimes to treat the patient, the tumor must be treated. Just because drugs or treatment options are available, however, does not mean they should be offered to all patients. If the treatment is worse than the disease or the patient's performance status is poor, tumor-shrinking therapy may offer little for the patient. There are always other options for patients—to treat the symptoms, the side effects, and the pain often associated with advanced cancer.

—*Partial response* means shrinkage of the tumor or the total amount of disease by greater than 50 percent. If a tumor shrinks greater than 50 percent but does not completely disappear, this indicates that therapy can possibly control the disease and patients may live a longer and better life but are unlikely to be cured. Obviously, the greater the amount of tumor shrinkage, the better. Patients with significant clinical symptoms may benefit if the tumor shrinkage correlates with improvement of symptoms—that is, if patients experience less pain, a decrease in swelling of the legs, or less bleeding from the bladder.

—*Performance status* is basically how you are doing. Study after study in cancer care has demonstrated that the best predictor of how a patient will do with therapy is how the patient is doing before the therapy begins, or at what level he or she is functioning. Cancer can cause many symptoms that affect and possibly slow a patient's ability to attend to normal daily activities. To assess a patient's performance status, the doctor asks questions about level of activity, time spent in bed or resting, ability to perform normal chores, or which chores cannot be carried out.

Patients with significantly impaired performance status—for example, those who are in bed more than half the day or require assistance with most activities of daily living—may not be good candidates for chemotherapy. They often have more side effects and less tumor responses to therapy compared to more active patients. Patients with excellent performance status often tolerate the therapy well but can become frustrated because their level of activity is slowed by the therapy.

—*Progressive disease* is the appearance of new lesions, the worsening or increasing of symptoms attributable to the tumor, or an increase in the size of the tumor greater than 25 percent. There are few, if any, reasons to continue a therapy if the tumor continues to grow while on that therapy. That particular therapy should be stopped and, if the person is still well (with a good performance status), another form of therapy can be offered.

—*Response* refers to the way a tumor reacts to therapy.

—*Stable disease* is defined as no real change in the size of the tumor. Medically, tumors can change by 25 percent—either growing or shrinking—and still be considered stable. A minor response may translate into improvement in symptoms. However, if a person suffers a great deal from chemotherapy and the disease remains stable or slowly progresses, then it is probably best that the therapy be stopped, as the risks seem to be outweighing the benefits. On the other hand, if the tumor had been growing before the start of therapy and the therapy is tolerated well, stable disease may be a favorable outcome and more of the same therapy should be offered. A good working relationship with your physician is important in making decisions involving these issues.

Uses for Chemotherapy

As the definitions above indicate, chemotherapy is used in a number of different contexts to treat bladder cancer. For superficial bladder cancer, intravesicle therapy is sometimes prescribed. This refers to treating the inside of the bladder with a chemotherapeutic agent. (See chapter 4 for a more complete discussion of intravesicle therapy.)

Chemotherapy for muscle-invasive bladder cancer is classified by five different categories:

—preoperative, or neoadjuvant
—postoperative, or adjuvant
—high risk for relapse
—locally advanced or positive nodes
—metastatic bladder cancer

How Chemotherapy Works

Cancer is a disease of altered cell growth. A bladder cell that has become malignant possesses two qualities that distinguish it as cancer:

—Unlimited, uncontrolled growth and proliferation. Proliferation results when cells lose the ability to die and pile up instead of making way for new cells.
—The ability to metastasize, or spread. Benign tumors may grow in one place but not qualify as cancer because they do not have the capability to spread to other areas.

The first chemotherapy drugs attacked growing cancer cells. For cell growth, a cell must constantly duplicate its DNA to pass on to its offspring after division. A cell preparing to divide is like a very busy factory with a production deadline rapidly approaching. Chemotherapy drugs have been designed to attack the DNA so that the offspring cells receive ineffective copies of the DNA, causing them to die. Other drugs gum up the machinery needed to divide, like an equipment malfunction. Newer drugs actually trigger pathways in cells unable to die which activate internal "suicide" molecules that the cell had forgotten how to produce. All of these drugs have the goal of making it harder for the cancer cell to survive, proliferate, and spread.

These cell-killing strategies attack dividing or growing cells, but they are not truly specific to cancer and can also affect healthy cells. However, only a few types of cells in our bodies are constantly replenishing themselves the way cancer cells are. The cells of our hair, cells in the lining of our intestines, and blood cells made in the bone marrow are the few types of cells that are growing and turning over regularly. Chemotherapy often affects these cells as well as the rapidly multiplying cancer cells. That is why people having chemotherapy often experience hair loss, loose stool or diarrhea, and low blood counts (which put chemotherapy patients at risk for infection, bleeding, or anemia). Our normal tissues recover quickly and, because they are healthy, are rarely permanently damaged by the chemotherapy. Cancer cells often do not have the mechanisms to repair themselves, so cancer deposits shrink or stop growing in response to therapy, while the normal cells of the body recover.

Unfortunately, tumor cells can become resistant to the effects of chemotherapy. Sometimes cancer cells develop mechanisms to block the effect of chemotherapy. Chemotherapy needs to get into the cancer cell to kill it. Once inside the cell, the drug takes a little while to deliver its punch. Some cancer cells develop a sort of pump to get rid of the chemotherapy drugs, removing them before they have a chance to kill the cell. Another reason for resistance to or ineffectiveness of chemotherapy drugs is inadequate blood supply to the area of the tumor. If blood supply is poor or restricted, then the drug may not be able get near the cancer cell. In some cases, the cancer is not actively growing and, since the drugs only work when the cancer cell is dividing, treatment is not effective. Because of these factors, chemotherapy is often repeated at different times, in an effort to "outsmart" the cancer cells.

The effects of chemotherapy on the immune system are unclear. Certainly the white blood cells, which are responsible for our immune system, are often temporarily harmed by chemotherapy. The number of white blood cells drops very low after treatment with many chemotherapy regimens. Because of this, the patient is at high risk of developing a life-threatening infection right after treatment. With prompt use of antibiotics, observation for any signs of infections, and sometimes white cell growth factor support (administration of a drug called GMCSF, which stimulates the bone marrow), the real risk of a serious infection can be greatly lowered.

The long-term effects of chemotherapy on the immune system appear to be minimal. Patients are not required to have their immunizations repeated, for example, because the immune system retains enough "memory"

of immunization to continue to prevent those infections. Patients sometimes ask us whether the effects of chemotherapy on the immune system
might allow the cancer to grow. They wonder whether the immune system
has been helping to keep the cancer in check. Although little scientific
evidence exists to support this point, there *is* considerable evidence that
chemotherapy has cured people of their disease, in cancers such as testicu-
lar cancer, lymphomas, and bladder cancer. Also, recent findings suggest
that chemotherapy may *activate* the immune system's response to cancer
cells. Researchers have shown that cancer can grow unchecked in patients
because their immune system does not recognize that a cancer exists—it
looks too much like normal tissue for the immune system to want to eliminate it. In some cases, chemotherapy may stimulate the immune system by
alerting it to the presence of cancer. A cancer cell that is being killed
by chemotherapy may look suspicious to the immune system, triggering a
hypervigilant response to remaining cancer cells and prompting a partner-
ship between the immune system and the chemotherapy to eradicate
cancer.

As noted earlier, often chemotherapy treatments consist of a combination of drugs to attack the cancer. Drugs with different mechanisms of action cause different side effects and generate different cancer resistance
mechanisms. With combination strategies, the cancer cell is attacked
through multiple routes, increasing the chance of wiping it out. One agent
may affect the lining of the intestines more than another agent, while another agent may affect the bone marrow without altering the intestine
lining. One drug may be quickly pumped out of the cancer cell, whereas
another might not. Our knowledge of drug activity, side effects, and resistance mechanisms is used to improve combination therapies for bladder
cancer.

Drugs Used to Treat Bladder Cancer

Now that we have discussed how chemotherapy works and why and when
it is used, let's take a look at some of the specific drugs we're talking about.
Chemotherapeutic drugs are used alone and in combination to treat bladder cancer. In this section, we list the individual drugs most commonly

used to treat bladder cancer and describe how each works, how it will be administered, and what side effects can be expected.

Cisplatinum

Studies show us that cisplatinum is one of the most active drugs available in the treatment of bladder cancer, especially when combined with other drugs. Used alone, it shrinks tumors 12 percent of the time—not as high a rate as some other drugs when used alone—but when other chemo drugs are combined with cisplatinum, cisplatinum increases the effectiveness of those other drugs. Cisplatinum, in combination with other drugs, is the standard first-line treatment regimen for bladder cancer. It is most often combined with methotrexate, vinblastine, and adriamycin, in the four-drug regimen known as M-VAC, or with paclitaxel or gemcitabine.

Cisplatinum, a heavy metal, works by binding with the DNA of cancer cells and thereby inflicting irreversible damage on it. The cancer cell is unable to remove the platinum from its DNA and dies because it can no longer use its DNA. Cisplatinum is given by intravenous infusion. Researchers are looking into the effectiveness of administering platinum-based drugs orally, but the drug in this form is not yet readily available outside of a clinical trial.

When cisplatinum was first developed, it was nearly shelved because it was thought to be too toxic. Now it is one of the most commonly used chemotherapy agents for all of cancer therapy. It does cause severe nausea and vomiting, but we have found that these symptoms can be considerably lessened or alleviated if patients take antinausea medicines before, during, and after therapy with cisplatinum. In fact, a whole pharmaceutical industry has been created to develop drugs that curtail cisplatinum-induced nausea. Drugs like ondansetron and granisetron have greatly reduced the nausea and vomiting associated with cisplatinum.

Another effect of cisplatinum's toxicity is evident in the kidneys. As a heavy metal, cisplatinum can settle in the tubules of the kidney, making them sluggish and unable to clear normal bodily wastes. To try to prevent this, we give patients intravenous fluids containing salt or diuretics ("water pills"), which increase the kidneys' flow rates and urine output. Increasing the flow of fluid through the kidneys helps to wash out the cisplatinum.

Patients with renal failure may receive a reduced dose or a different drug if lowered kidney function makes it impossible to use cisplatinum safely.

For some patients, the amount of fluid required to hydrate them in anticipation of the cisplatinum may be too much for their hearts or lungs to handle. Close observation is required in patients who have weak or frail hearts. Some patients are brought into the hospital to make sure the extra fluid is adequately tolerated. Also, if treatment requires higher doses of cisplatinum, these are often administered in the hospital.

Cisplatinum can affect hearing and the nerves of the hands and feet. As a heavy metal, it can deposit in the small nerves, particularly at the tips of the fingers and toes. The body can sometimes repair this nerve damage, or neuropathy, but in many cases it is permanent. In your follow-up care after chemotherapy, your physician will ask you questions and examine you regarding these symptoms, if they occur. Patients most often describe the symptoms as numbness or tingling at the fingertips or feet. Certain drug combinations, such as using cisplatinum with vincristine or paclitaxel, may increase the likelihood of this complication.

Cisplatinum can also affect the bone marrow, resulting in a decline of white cell, platelet, and red cell counts. The white cells and platelets recover within ten to fourteen days after the therapy. Other, less common side effects include change in taste and hair loss.

Cisplatinum is an excellent radiation sensitizer, acting to make radiation work better. It is often used in combination with radiation to increase the efficacy of the radiation (see chapter 7).

Carboplatinum

Carboplatinum is closely related to cisplatinum. In formulating carboplatinum, changes were made in the structure of cisplatinum to cause less nausea and fewer associated kidney effects. Its effectiveness is comparable to that of cisplatinum if given at the appropriate doses. In direct comparison, cisplatinum seems to have greater activity than carboplatinum, which is why it is the drug used in most combination regimens.

Carboplatinum is given intravenously. It does not require intensive fluid hydration prior to administration and is almost always given on an outpatient basis. It does induce nausea, but to a lesser extent than cisplatinum. It also affects peripheral or distant nerves less than cisplatinum does. Carboplatinum has a greater effect on platelets than does cisplatinum. Otherwise, the two drugs are comparable.

Methotrexate

Methotrexate was one of the first chemotherapy drugs developed to fight cancer. It is now also commonly used to treat rheumatologic disorders such as rheumatoid arthritis, lupus, and psoriasis. Methotrexate affects DNA synthesis by making the building blocks unavailable to the cell. It is routinely administered intravenously. The drug affects rapidly proliferating cells, so hair loss is common, as are sores or ulcers in the mouth, and loose stools or diarrhea are possible as well. Methotrexate can also affect bone marrow cells. It is not used in patients who have a problem with collection of fluid, such as fluid in the lungs or a pleural effusion. Methotrexate is often used to treat tumors that have spread to the brain or the fluid surrounding the brain. For bladder cancer, it is often used in combination with cisplatinum, vinblastine, and adriamycin.

Piritrexim

Piritrexim is a new chemotherapy agent currently under clinical investigation. It acts similarly to methotrexate but seems to have fewer side effects. It has not yet been approved for use in bladder cancer, and it is given orally.

Vinblastine

Vinblastine is a chemotherapy agent derived from the periwinkle (vinca) flower. It inhibits the formation of the wiring within the cell required for cell division. The scaffolding on which the DNA separates is called the mitotic spindle. Vinblastine and a closely related compound, vincristine, inhibit the mitotic spindle, preventing cell duplication. Its side effects are few. It can cause mild nausea, but its greatest effects are on the bone marrow cells. Vinblastine can have some effect on peripheral nerves, though a greater effect is associated with vincristine. Vinblastine is administered intravenously; this should be done with care so that it does not spill from the vein, because it can cause damage to surrounding tissue if it leaks during administration.

Adriamycin

Adriamycin is a topoisomerase II inhibitor. Topoisomerase II is an enzyme involved in replication of DNA; this enzyme helps the DNA unwind to duplicate itself. By inhibiting this interaction, adriamycin damages DNA and promotes cell death. Adriamycin is commonly used in breast cancer therapy. In bladder cancer, it is often used in combination with other agents like cisplatinum, methotrexate, or vinblastine. It is administered intravenously and can be harmful to local skin tissues if it leaks during administration. Adriamycin causes little nausea, but mouth ulcers are often an unpleasant side effect. It also affects the bone marrow cells and hair follicles, but these effects are reversible—white blood cells replenish themselves, and hair grows back.

With chronic use, adriamycin can cause a weakening of the heart muscle. For the most part, effects on the heart are dose-dependent, that is, the chances of the heart being affected increase as the doses increase. The size of the doses used for bladder cancer rarely cause concern, but the effects on the heart still may occur in some bladder cancer patients treated with the drug. This complication is rare, but care is taken to prevent it. Often the oncologist will evaluate cardiac function with an echocardiogram or a nuclear medicine test to establish a baseline before or very soon after initiating therapy with adriamycin. These tests are noninvasive and may be repeated every couple of months during the course of therapy to rule out any decline in heart function.

Paclitaxel

Paclitaxel (Taxol) is a relative newcomer in the treatment of bladder cancer. It is derived from the bark of the Pacific yew tree and is commonly used in patients with breast and ovarian cancer. It inhibits cell division by binding to the mitotic spindles, gumming them up and disabling them during cell division. Paclitaxel is given intravenously over three to twenty-four hours every three weeks. Early studies suggested that the twenty-four-hour schedule was more effective than the three-hour schedule, but the three-hour schedule can be given in the clinic while the twenty-four-hour schedule requires hospitalization. Most regimens use the three-hour schedule.

Allergic reactions can occur with the administration of paclitaxel, so patients take premedications of dexamethasone (a steroid) the night before and the morning of therapy, then before therapy patients are given diphenhydramine (Benadryl) and either cimetidine (Tagamet), ranitidine (Zantac), or famotidine (Pepcid). These drugs work fairly well to eliminate allergic reactions.

Paclitaxel causes hair loss, bone and muscle aches, and drops in blood counts. A common side effect is asymptomatic slowing of the heart rate during administration. Paclitaxel can affect the peripheral nerves, causing a neuropathy of the hands and feet. The drug may also cause constipation if slowing of intestinal function occurs. Paclitaxel is associated with minimal nausea, and it can be administered as a single agent or in combination with cisplatinum or carboplatinum.

Gemcitabine

Gemcitabine (Gemzar) is another new drug that may prove useful in treating bladder cancer. It has been approved for use in patients with pancreatic cancer. Gemcitabine mimics a necessary building block of DNA, and, by fooling the DNA, the drug causes DNA damage that in turn causes cancer cell death.

Gemcitabine is administered intravenously once a week for three weeks, followed by a week without the drug. It is associated with minimal nausea and is given in the clinic. It may affect the bone marrow cells and may produce low-grade fevers, but it is very well tolerated in general. It is currently undergoing a clinical trial combining it with cisplatinum. These combination studies look extremely encouraging and show high response rates.

Ifosfamide

Ifosfamide binds with DNA, preventing replication. It is administered intravenously, most commonly by continuous infusions. It is associated with significant nausea, so antinausea medications are used during its administration. Ifosfamide can cause bleeding of the urinary bladder lining and is often administered with fluids containing salt and with MESNA, an agent that protects the bladder from the drug's harmful effects. Ifosfamide has profound effects on the bone marrow cells. It is often used in combination with vinblastine, gallium, or both. Because of its toxicity, it is often used after other regimens have failed. An older, similar drug, cyclophosphamide, is also sometimes used for advanced bladder cancer.

Gallium

Gallium is another metal that works against bladder cancer. It is not commonly used for bladder cancer because it has potentially serious side effects and few oncologists have experience with its use. Gallium can be used to treat high calcium levels associated with cancer, and it causes calcium declines in patients with normal calcium prior to therapy. It is administered intravenously and is given in the hospital for close observation. Gallium can also cause an inflammation of the nerves that supply the eye. It can be used as a single agent or in combination with agents like vinblastine or ifosfamide.

Putting It All Together

On your first visit to the medical oncologist, you may feel both anticipation and anxiety. You may feel that your whole life is in your oncologist's hands and that to survive you must do what he or she tells you to do. You may be concerned that the doctor is very busy and does not have time to go into the details that interest you and answer all of your many questions. These are normal feelings and should not get in the way of a satisfactory interaction with your doctor. You must ask questions! No question is a stupid question. If you don't get an answer, keep asking.

Often, the physician sees all that is happening to you as routine. While this may seem to trivialize what has no doubt become the most important thing in your life, it can also be comforting to you to know that what is happening to you has happened to others and that your doctor has been there and helped them. He or she has been down the treatment path with a large number of patients and knows where the bumps in the road are.

The course of treatment is not one straight path but a collection of approaches, each with differing benefits and risks. For the most part, you will have options regarding how to proceed with your therapy. Ask the doctor for alternatives, and ask him or her to discuss treatment options and explain the reason for his or her recommendations. Don't expect the doctor to make your treatment decisions for you. The better strategy is for you to make your own decisions based on your doctor's recommendations.

If you are going to receive chemotherapy, the nurses and the doctor should let you know when to expect side effects and what signs and symptoms to look for. Every drug regimen has its own quirks and things to watch out for. Follow-up and duration of treatment may also vary.

Sometimes it is helpful to talk to other people who have been through what awaits you. You can ask the doctor or nurse to put you in contact with patients who have received similar therapies. These veterans of chemotherapy may give you good advice and let you know how they felt. Yet remember that every patient is different, as is every individual's response. Support groups for patients with cancer are another resource to aid your journey through treatment. Studies even show that patients involved in support groups live longer than those who do not participate. However, support groups are not for everybody. Strong support at home, from family and friends, can be extremely important in helping you survive cancer.

We encourage you to get a second opinion to confirm the diagnosis and review treatment plans. (Not all insurance carriers cover second opinions, so those expenses may be out of your pocket.) Second opinions are helpful, although rarely do they change a plan of care. In many cases, they provide you with the opportunity to meet two different doctors and their staff. Your trust for and comfort with the physician who is caring for you is important to your cancer therapy. Second opinions give you the chance to be selective at a time when you otherwise may feel there are no options. One potential problem with second opinions is the time it might take to get one, when in some cases the speed of starting therapy may be the issue. You can ask the first doctor you see if this is a factor.

To Work or Not to Work?

Many patients ask whether they can work while on chemotherapy and if there are any limitations about being around other people during this time. Usually the decision to work is an individual one. There are many regimens and many individual responses to each regimen, and sometimes you will not be able to predict what you will be capable of until after you have begun the therapy.

Some regimens will allow you to continue to work, while others are more intense and exhausting. Because most cycles of a particular therapy are alike, you can see how the first cycle goes and determine for yourself whether or not you can continue to work. In many cases, time off from work to receive treatment is necessary. Hospitalization is required to receive some of the drugs. Other drugs can be administered in the clinic but need to be given with intravenous fluids that keep you out of work most of the day. Still other drugs can be given in fifteen minutes, and you can be back to work after a stop in the clinic.

Most of the regimens of drugs for bladder cancer decrease the white blood cell count and sometimes the platelet levels. A low white blood count means you are at risk of infection, so it's not a good idea to be around people who are sick or may be sick. Low platelet levels also put you at risk for bleeding, so some limitations are placed on physical activity to avoid injury. You may also feel tired and "wiped out" in the days after therapy, and this may prevent you from working or mean working shorter hours or resting when you get home from work.

Getting Chemotherapy: How It's Done

A typical chemotherapy day will vary, depending on whether you are admitted to the hospital for treatment or are receiving the therapy as an outpatient. In either case, if the drug is administered in the vein you will have an intravenous catheter placed in one of the veins of the arm or hand. Having the catheter inserted is similar to having your blood drawn with a needle, but the needle is replaced with a thin plastic tube that can stay in your vein while you are receiving the therapy. Nurses or phlebotomists usually put the catheters in and check to make sure there is a good flow of blood and none of the fluid leaks into the skin.

The chemotherapy drug is infused directly into the vein through the catheter's plastic tubing. This should not hurt unless the chemical is leaking or the drug is given faster than recommended. After the drug and any accompanying fluid or medications are given, the catheter is removed and you can go home. Depending on how likely it is that the chemotherapy drug will cause nausea, you will be given medications to prevent and control the nausea. Some medications, like paclitaxel (Taxol), require premedication with steroids and antihistamine drugs such as diphenhydramine (Benadryl). Many of the drugs given to reduce side effects are sedating, so you must have someone with you to drive you home. Once you have gone through a cycle or two of chemotherapy, you will become more knowledgeable about how you tolerate therapy and what you can and cannot do.

Some patients choose to have a more permanent venous access device placed so they do not have to get stuck and have a new catheter put in for each treatment. Factors affecting this decision include how easy it is to access your veins and how many treatments you will be having. These more permanent catheters come in various forms and are placed into one of the bigger veins in your body. The simplest, a peripherally inserted central catheter (or PICC catheter), is placed in the big vein at the crease of your elbow. From there, a long plastic tube is threaded into the veins in your chest above your heart. Specialized nurses or doctors put these catheters in, and they may not be available at all hospitals.

More commonly used catheters for the large veins are placed under the collarbone and tunneled under the skin. These catheters can stay in a long time and can be used to draw blood as well as to administer chemotherapy or fluids. They are usually placed by surgeons or interventional radiologists. If you receive one, you will be taught how to care for the catheter at home. For the most part, this simply involves flushing the tubing every day to keep it from becoming blocked.

One final type of venous access device is a port or reservoir that is buried under the skin. The port has a soft spot, into which needles are placed to draw blood or to administer therapy. Surgeons typically place these ports, and they have to be flushed by trained personnel at the clinic during your visits. Talk with your doctor or the nurse who administers your therapy as to which catheter may be best for you. The risks associated with all these central venous access devices are infection and clotting. You will be taught how to look for early signs of these problems.

Taking Care of Yourself

Maintaining a well-balanced diet and keeping up with a simple exercise routine are an important part of your care plan. Nutrition and exercise are complementary to your therapy and should be maintained even after the therapy has been completed. Early in your therapy, a visit with a nutritionist may be helpful to plan a program specific to your food likes and dislikes. Therapy may change your sense of taste, however, and foods you liked in the past may no longer be appealing to you. Likewise, you may develop new tastes.

Taking vitamins may help you maintain your strength, particularly if you take in less food and calories because of therapy. Some vitamins have cancer-fighting properties, but not all can be recommended. Antioxidants like vitamin E and beta carotene have received a great deal of media attention, but the jury is still out on the role of vitamins in patients who have been diagnosed with cancer. Most of the studies that have been done on vitamins are in the area of cancer prevention. Many of these vitamin regimens are also expensive and can significantly alter your lifestyle.

A vegetarian diet is another dietary alternative that may appeal to some patients. Any changes in diet, vitamin, and exercise routine should be reviewed with your doctor. Some doctors may not immediately talk with you about nutrition and diet, but it is an important subject to bring up with them anyway. There is little proof that these therapies are beneficial, but most have few harmful side effects. You can find out more information about these types of complementary therapies from your doctor or nurse or through reading at the library or on the Internet.

If you are considering changing your diet, using vitamins, or changing your lifestyle, be honest with yourself about why you are making these changes. If you are doing it only to get rid of your cancer and the cancer grows, then these changes are not working. If you are doing it to feel better and you do feel better, then keep it up. Unless you know why you are doing something and can assess whether you are achieving your goals, you can spend a lot of time and effort on these alternatives with seemingly little effect. To make an analogy, your doctor will discontinue a chemotherapy regimen if it is not working and will continue a therapy if it is—that is, if it is shrinking your tumor or you are having a clinical response as measured by an improvement in pain.

Getting on Top of Side Effects

As we have seen, the chemotherapy drugs that attack the cancer cells in your body pack a powerful punch that can be felt in many different systems, at different times, and with varying durations and degrees of intensity. When you receive therapy, the doctors will break down your side effects into those that occur with or shortly after receiving the therapy and those that are late effects of the therapy.

To summarize the discussion earlier in this chapter: acute, or early, side effects include:

—nausea and vomiting
—fatigue
—weight loss
—lack of appetite
—hair loss
—drops in blood counts

You will be instructed about what to do when these problems arise and who to contact. (If you do not receive this information, ask.) You will be given medications to take home to combat the side effects. You are likely to have clinical follow-up in the week or so after your therapy to update your blood counts. If your blood counts drop, your doctor will explain whether this means any limitations are necessary. In some cases, if counts drop below a certain level, you may need to be hospitalized so intravenous antibiotics can be administered to prevent any infection from setting in while your immune system is compromised.

Acute effects usually resolve a week or so before the next scheduled treatment. So you will often start feeling better again soon before you have to repeat the therapy—not much fun, but you will learn to accept this as the pattern of your life for a period. Most acute effects are readily reversible once the drugs have been discontinued. Severer side effects may suggest to your doctor that a change in therapy or a change in dose is needed. If your doctor does reduce your dose because of side effects, he or she is doing it for your safety. The positive side of this is that if the drug is making you so sick that the dose needs to be reduced, it is likely your tumor is also seeing a lot of the drug. A dose reduction does not translate into smaller tumor responses, but this does not mean your doctor should start you out with smaller doses. The doses chosen at the start of therapy are the ones that experience has shown us are most likely to work. From this starting point, most regimens can then be tailored to fit the individual patient, based on side effects.

Late effects of therapy include:

—chronic anemias
—sterility or infertility
—nerve damage
—peripheral neuropathy
—new cancer caused by the therapy you received to get rid of your diagnosed cancer

Chemotherapy given over months, which is the normal routine, can create all of these problems. The anemias will usually resolve over time, but you could need blood transfusions or growth factor shots to help your red cells come back. All of the regimens can have effects on unborn children, so adequate birth control, if appropriate, is needed while receiving therapy. Men may consider banking sperm if they know or think they will wish to father children after treatment. Women should consult with their gynecologist about issues related to chemotherapy's side effects. Menstrual periods may become irregular or cease altogether. If a woman does become pregnant while on therapy, she should talk with her doctor about the implications and discuss available options.

The peripheral neuropathy may reverse slowly or change from a numbness to a fiery pain as the nerves regenerate. The neuropathy may be worse in patients prone to neuropathies that are not chemotherapy related, like those due to diabetes or chronic alcohol use. There are a few drugs that may help manage these side effects if they are severe.

Though it rarely happens, the chemotherapy you receive may cause another cancer. This ironic side effect is important to hear at the start, particularly if it is thought that your tumor is curable. The risk of second malignancies is less than 2 percent of all patients. Even after you have completed your therapy, continue to see your oncologist, who can be on guard to catch these second cancers early. When making decisions about chemotherapy, you may feel that you have only bad choices—what cures this cancer may have the chance of giving you another cancer. However, if you are being offered chemotherapy it is because your oncologist thinks the benefits far outweigh the risks.

The decision to stop a therapy is based on how you and your tumor respond to it. If the therapy is working and you remain well, you can continue therapy for many months. Often a predetermined number of treatments is planned at the beginning, and after this number has been completed the treatment is stopped. Other doctors stop therapy two cycles after the treatment has worked completely or once the tumor has become stable and is not shrinking anymore.

If the therapy is not working, as judged by an increase in the size of tumor or by increasing symptoms, your therapy should be discontinued and alternatives should be discussed. If your cancer shrinks and then remains stable or stops growing while on therapy but does not shrink further, the decision to stop therapy is often a joint decision between you and your doctor. Some people are frightened to stop therapy if the tumor has not completely disappeared, thinking that the chemotherapy has been keeping the tumor in check. Some doctors will continue therapy as long as it is not hurting you, while others would discontinue the therapy and watch you. If the tumor grows back after the therapy is stopped, this suggests that you should be on a new therapy or, if it has been a long time since your original treatment, that you should use the previous regimen.

Once you have completed a therapy, you will still continue to see your oncologist frequently, scheduling visits three or four times a year. Scans or x-rays will be taken to check for recurrences. If you have new or recurring symptoms between scheduled office visits, call your doctor. Some patients experience anxiety at the end of therapy when the doctor arranges follow-up in three months. You have been seeing the doctor frequently when on therapy, and there is often a certain comfort in seeing your doctor on a regular basis. But remember, the reason you underwent therapy was so you could eventually stay away from doctors, to get on with your life. Hopefully this will become an actuality for everyone reading this. However, the reality of living with cancer is the fear of its return or its causing an early death. Sometimes the cancer is bigger than all of us. It is not your fault if the treatment for your cancer does not work, nor is it the fault of those treating you. The experience of living with and surviving cancer is a tough road, but more and more patients are successfully getting down the road alive and well.

CHAPTER NINE

Some Advice from Our Patients

A diagnosis of bladder cancer greatly affects all who get the disease, both mentally and physically. Many patients have told us that almost every aspect of their lives changed after their diagnosis. But learning to live with bladder cancer, while extraordinarily challenging, is not impossible. Talking to bladder cancer patients and asking them how they have handled life with this disease, we have compiled a list of seven of their recommendations to help others better cope with their disease.

Share Your Concerns

Friends and family can be your most valuable source of emotional support. Don't underestimate the value of just sitting down and talking with someone who cares for you.

Learning that you have bladder cancer can be devastating—many patients have told us that. Reactions to the diagnosis can range from denial to fear, anger to depression. We hear many common emotional themes: "It can't be! You've made a mistake!" "I'm afraid of the unknown and the uncertainty of dying." "God can't do this to me." "Why me?" "What's the use in living?" In some instances, the shock from hearing the diagnosis causes patients to experience actual physical symptoms: chills, dizziness, disorientation, nausea, and loss of appetite. These are all normal reactions, but they may be very difficult to handle in a rational manner.

Being able to talk openly about your feelings, experiences, and apprehensions with those who care can help you cope with the disease and its uncertainties. Many patients have told us that the ability to tell others about their hopes, fears, needs, and wants is invaluable. "I just can't express how important that is," we have heard from patient after patient. Or: "Talking with others helps to allow the practical side to set in, and time to gather the forces to lick this disease."

Coping with the diagnosis of bladder cancer begins with the decision to accept it and build upon a positive attitude. Patients emphasize the need to maintain a positive attitude and overcome any fatalistic ideas. They tell us: "You can't look back to why did it happen, because it did happen. It's here!" or "You need to accept the fact that you have bladder cancer, and concentrate on what you are going to do about it. Survival should be your main goal."

Get as Much Information as You Can

Have your physician or oncologist explain the implications of a diagnosis of bladder cancer and what it means to you. A well-informed patient usually does better in many ways than an uninformed patient. You can only maintain control and make wise decisions if you have the facts and can compare the various options. Questions you may want to ask include:

1. What is bladder cancer?
2. Is it curable?
3. How long do I have to live?
4. How bad is my disease?
5. What do I do now?
6. Are there tests that I need to undergo?
7. What are my treatment options?
8. What are the risks and benefits?
9. Will I need a urostomy?
10. Will my sex life change?
11. Will I need to change my normal activities?
12. How often do I need check-ups?
13. Who can I go to for a second opinion?

Many patients recommend writing down your questions as you think of them and then taking notes or bringing a tape recorder on your doctors' visits. Some patients add that bringing a relative or a close friend to the visit, to help listen and take notes, is also helpful. A common theme expressed by patients is, "Sometimes, it's better to have an extra ear along, because the information is so overwhelming."

You may have concerns about the future and your family, as well as about the overall cost of your medical care. Nurses, social workers, and financial counselors are helpful with these concerns. Other sources of information include the public library, the Cancer Information Service network, the American Cancer Society, the American Foundation for Urologic Disease, the United Ostomy Association, the Physicians Data Query, and other support groups.

> Be sure to ask for clarification on anything that is not clear.
>
> Don't be shy or feel guilty about taking up your doctor's time.
>
> Remember, no question is foolish.

Find Out What to Expect in the Way of Testing

Inquire about the tests you will need to undergo to allow your doctor to determine the extent of your disease. Don't hesitate to ask "What's it like?" or "What are the risks of undergoing the procedure?" or "What can be done if I choose not to undergo the procedure?" Also, you may want to ask for names of other patients who are willing to share information about their experiences regarding tests and procedures. Remember, though, that each individual has his or her own reaction to procedures.

As you read in chapter 2, tests that you may be asked to undergo include IVP (intravenous pyelogram), cystoscopy, CAT scan, bone scan, and MRI (magnetic resonance imaging). An intravenous pyelogram is a test that allows your doctor to examine your kidneys, ureter, and bladder. Some patients find this test was "not uncomfortable at all"; others, however, state that they experienced a feeling of warmth, nausea, dizziness, or some discomfort from the dye given for this procedure. A cystoscopy is a procedure that allows your doctor to examine your bladder. Some patients have stated that this procedure can be uncomfortable and "not a very pleasant experience." Others have said, "It's not as bad as I imagined." One patient suggested that "remaining relaxed is the key to avoiding much discomfort, and you need to ask your doctor to prescribe medication to help you relax if you can't do it on your own."

Your doctor may order a CAT scan and bone scan to further evaluate your disease. Both of these tests are painless. In preparation for these tests, you will be asked to drink several ounces of contrast dye and also receive an IV injection of dye. One patient stated, "If you're not used to drinking large quantities of liquids, this is a bit difficult, but nothing that I couldn't overcome." You are asked to lie on a narrow table, which moves you automatically through a scanning ring while a computer turns your x-rays into three-dimensional pictures. This can be unsettling, because you will hear the sounds of motors and gears as the scanner takes a series of pictures. Another test your doctor may order is an MRI, which will produce more detailed pictures than the CAT scan. MRI scanning is also painless, but it can be much noisier than the CAT scanner and requires that you be placed in a tubular chamber that is only open at one end. If you are claustrophobic, ask for an eye covering or a mild sedative to help you relax.

Find an Expert to Treat Your Disease

Seek a physician or oncologist who specializes in bladder cancer. A doctor in whom you have confidence will assure you the best possible care. "Your physician is someone who will support your strengths and hopes," patients tell us, "so you need to trust him or her."

Patients also emphasize to us the importance of getting a second opinion about a diagnosis and treatment plan prior to consenting to any type of major medical treatment. With a diagnosis as serious as bladder cancer, you need reassurance that you are doing the best thing possible for the treatment of your disease. Physicians or oncologists who offer second opinions about your diagnosis and treatment options can be found through various channels, such as: (1) the Cancer Information Service, at 1-800-4-CANCER, (2) the National Cancer Institute's designated cancer centers, (3) the American Cancer Society, (4) a nearby hospital, or (5) your own physician or oncologist. You may wish to ask other bladder cancer patients for the names of doctors who can give second opinions. If you are not confident with the second opinion, seek a third opinion. A recurrent theme expressed by patients is, "It's your life!"

Get Details about Treatment Effects and Side Effects

Inquire about the specifics of treatments and what the potential side effects from therapy can be. The important thing for you is to know what to expect. A good starting point is reading chapters 5 through 8 in this book for explanations of treatment details. Understanding the fundamentals of each type of treatment procedure will give you a platform on which to build your knowledge. For example, you might know that surgery involves removing the cancer and any involved organs, but you may not know that this treatment necessitates a short hospital stay and approximately six to eight weeks of convalescence (if there are no complications).

Patients are often well informed about some aspects of chemotherapy, including the way drugs work, how they are given, and potential side effects. But you may not be as well informed about the details of each particular regimen and the fact that each treatment session will usually include blood and urine work as well as a brief physical examination.

Patients usually know that radiation therapy involves the use of high-energy rays to shrink the tumor and destroy cancerous cells, but they may not realize that treatments are usually given once a day, Monday through Friday, for several weeks, and that while the radiation dose itself only lasts several minutes, the visit often takes longer.

Accounts from former patients are invaluable in learning what a treatment and its side effects will be like. Our patients offer advice like: "Try not to get discouraged, because you actually recover from most of the side effects from treatment," and "The treatments were brutal, but I got through them, and if I had to do it over again, I would."

Many patients are concerned about their sexuality as they go through treatment for bladder cancer and experience side effects and aftereffects. Discussing this issue with your partner, as well as with your physician, nurse, social worker, or other patients, can be helpful. One patient's advice summed up the feelings of many: "Though the physical act is often put on the back burner, your sexual expression is not. Your mental attitude can be a powerful force in overcoming any barriers that the diagnosis of bladder cancer has placed before you. Although there are many variables that can affect your sexual image, communicating your feelings to your partner can help cultivate a closeness that might not have developed otherwise."

Build a Support Network beyond Your Family

The sixth recommendation is to maintain a support system that includes people other than your family members. There are support groups composed of other bladder cancer patients—people who are facing problems like yours. Participation in a support group allows you to get a realistic picture of what to expect in the way of procedures, treatments, responses, and side effects. Sharing bladder cancer experiences with others also tends to help people better cope with the disease. Many patients tell us of the strength and encouragement they gain from the understanding of others who share what they are going through. Ask members of your health team to suggest groups that will help with emotional support, financial aid, transportation, home care, and rehabilitation.

Continue Follow-up Doctor Visits

Continue with close follow-ups with your physician, because bladder cancer can recur. To some people this is one of the most frustrating barriers to enjoying a happy life. Even when you are feeling strong and healthy, frequent visits to the doctor can be an unwanted reminder of the serious disease you've dealt with. It's normal for you to continue to have thoughts like, "Although I'm free of cancer, I'm not free of cancer" and "Has it returned?" or "Is it getting worse?" We have learned from our patients that life after bladder cancer, even with its uncertainties, can be good. Generally, we find recovering and recovered patients have a positive outlook.

Many patients have told us that counseling, participation in self-help groups, relaxation, and meditation were all beneficial. But overall, many of the patients indicated that as time goes on, so does the challenge.

All the recommendations above imply a potent mind-body connection, which many of our patients tell us is necessary if one is to survive this disease. Remember that the prospect for complete recovery from early bladder cancer is very good. As research continues to find better ways to treat this disease, the chances for cure and remission improve.

> Why worry? You can't let the disease ruin what life you have left. It can be high-quality time if you let it. Close monitoring gives you some peace of mind, just knowing that if it returns you have a chance of nipping it in the bud. And that's enough. What more can you do? The rest is up to God.

Research about bladder cancer diagnosis and treatment is being conducted all across the country. Much information comes from clinical trials of the National Cancer Institute, one of the major government-funded research centers. When laboratory research shows that a new treatment method has promise, it is used to treat cancer patients in clinical trials. These trials, as explained in chapter 8, are designed to answer scientific questions and evaluate the safety and effectiveness of treatment. At some point, if you are not getting the results you would hope for from conventional treatment, you may wish to participate in a clinical trial. It is important to understand your own objectives before participating in a trial. Ask yourself: Can the treatment give me what I'm are looking for? Can I hope for cure or remission? Will it give me relief from my symptoms or will it cause worse side effects? If this is the avenue you wish to pursue, the general consensus from our patients is, "Do it!"

Learning to live with a diagnosis of bladder cancer can be made easier by following the recommendations of others who have gone through it.

You need to adapt to the changes that accompany the diagnosis and not let the disease take over your life. To recap, you need to:

—Talk to those who care about you. Do not isolate yourself.
—Keep reading and researching.
—Talk to others with bladder cancer.
—Inquire about the implications of the diagnosis of bladder cancer (i.e., definition, prognosis, tests, procedures, treatments, follow-up).
—Trust: Choose a physician in whom you have confidence.
—Have patience and maintain close follow-up with your doctor.
—Hope: Maintain a positive attitude.

Anterior exenteration: the standard operation to remove the bladder in female patients, which involves not only the removal of the bladder and urethra but also the removal of the uterus, cervix, ovaries, and the anterior or front wall of the vagina. This operation has recently been modified so the urethra can be preserved. In addition, patients of childbearing age may wish to discuss with their surgeon techniques for preserving the uterus and cervix during cystectomy.

Biopsy: a procedure whereby a small piece of tissue is removed for analysis in the pathology laboratory, where the pathologist processes and examines the tissue under the microscope to evaluate the material for the presence of cancer cells. In addition to determining whether cancer is present, biopsies permit the pathologist to determine the depth of cancer penetration into the tissue in question.

Bladder: a muscular container that stores urine, located in the pelvis. The bladder has a thick wall, with a delicate interior lining, from which bladder cancers develop, and a heavy coat of fat on the outside. The bladder normally can hold about 400 to 500 cc of urine.

CAT scan: a specialized type of x-ray study in which complex imaging of the internal organs of the body permits evaluation for the presence of cancer and other abnormalities.

Chromosomes: collections of genes, which are made up of DNA. The normal human cell has 23 pairs of chromosomes. These provide a convenient way for cells to carry large numbers of genes around.

Colon: another name for the large intestine.

Continence: the ability to control the flow of urine from the bladder to the outside of the body. This capability is normally due to muscular structures called sphincters, which wrap around the base of the bladder and urethra. Removal of or damage to the urinary sphincters can result in an inability to control the flow of urine normally.

Continent catheterizable reconstruction: one of a group of internal reservoirs or new bladders (neobladders) that are not attached to the urethra. Instead, it is emptied through catheterization, usually through a special attachment to the skin that is similar to but smaller than the stoma for an ileal conduit. Continent reconstructions are often referred to by names given to them at the institution where the particular type of reconstruction was developed.

Cystoscope: a specialized instrument used by a physician to examine the interior of the urethra and a bladder. Cystoscopes come in many different shapes and sizes, and the latest models are small and flexible. Fiber optics has permitted the construction of delicate scopes that can be inserted into the urethra with minimum discomfort to the patient. The newer scopes allow excellent illumination of the interior of the urinary tract, permitting good visualization of the entire lining of the bladder. Some cystoscopes can take pictures and movies while the urologist views the urinary tract for documentation, the planning of therapy, and teaching.

Cystoscopy: A viewing procedure using a cystoscope.

DNA: deoxyribonucleic acid, molecules that are called the building blocks of life. These special chemicals, when arranged in their "normal" configuration, carry information that the cell needs in order to perform normal activities. When a chemical or group of chemicals in the DNA is damaged or altered in some way, mutations or structural alterations occur and can result in changes in the way normal cells grow. Certain alterations give rise to cancers and other specific diseases.

Enterostomal therapy: a branch of nursing devoted to the care of patients with various types of stomas.

Frozen section analysis: an immediate evaluation of biopsy material made possible by freezing the tissue in liquid nitrogen for rapid staining and evaluation under the microscope. While the preservation of tissue using this technique is not quite as good as when tissue is fixed using traditional chemical methods, sufficient information can be gathered to permit the pathologist to make an immediate diagnosis when necessary.

Gene: a special piece of DNA that directs a specific function in the normal human cell. When a gene is damaged in some way, the normal function that the gene performs may also be altered. Sometimes this results in the development of a specific disease, such as cancer.

Grade: a number describing the appearance of individual cells under the microscope. Grading of bladder tumors, usually on a scale of 1 to 3, is used to indicate the aggressiveness of individual tumor cells and is based on well-described criteria that pathologists employ in evaluating tissue specimens. Grade, simply stated, is the appearance of tumors under the microscope.

Hematuria: blood in the urine. Hematuria is either gross, meaning that the blood can be seen with the naked eye, or microscopic, meaning that blood can only be detected in the urine if the urine is examined under a microscope.

Ileal conduit: a simple form of urinary tract reconstruction which utilizes a small piece of intestine called the ileum. The ureters are implanted into this small segment of intestine, one end is closed with sutures, and the other is brought out to the skin to create a small opening, or mouth, called a stoma. Urine drains into a small pouch that fits over the stoma and attaches to the skin with an adhesive.

Intravenous pyelogram (IVP): a specialized x-ray that images the upper urinary tract. After the administration of intravenous contrast material, plain x-rays permit the visualization of the kidneys, the renal pelves, and the ureters. While excellent for looking at the upper urinary tract, this test is not particularly good for looking at the lower urinary tract. To examine the bladder comprehensively, doctors must perform cystoscopy.

Intravesical therapy: therapy delivered through a catheter inside the bladder, usually in the form of a chemical or drug. *Intravesical* simply means inside the bladder. A variety of different substances have been successfully used to treat the inside of the bladder to reduce the likelihood of bladder cancer recurrence.

Invasive bladder cancer: a bladder cancer that, in contrast to superficial cancers, invades the structures that lie beneath the lining cells. These tumors have characteristically bad biological behavior and are capable of spreading to other parts of the body without much warning. Accordingly, physicians are constantly on the lookout for evidence of disease spread in patients with invasive bladder carcinomas. Invasive cancers are less common than superficial ones, but they unfortunately spread to other parts of the body in about half of the patients who have this invasive disease.

Kidneys: paired organs located in the upper part of the abdomen behind the intestines, which are responsible for filtering waste material from blood and creating urine.

Lamina propria: a specialized layer of blood vessels and cells that separates the transitional epithelium from the actual muscle wall of the bladder.

Medical oncologist: a physician specializing in the treatment of cancer using medicines that are customarily administered intravenously.

Oncogene: a specific type of cancer-causing gene which, when it mutates, leads to abnormal stimulation of cell growth.

Neobladder: a new bladder usually constructed out of a piece of intestine and attached to the urethra. This is placed in the position that had been occupied by the bladder before it was removed because of disease.

p53: a particularly notable tumor-suppressor gene that is thought to play a central role in normal cells' growth regulation. Mutation of the p53 tumor suppressor gene has been shown to occur in up to 40 percent of invasive bladder carcinomas. Some scientists believe that p53 mutation may be a marker of the presence of a dangerous type of tumor which could require multiple therapies to cure.

Radiation oncologist: a physician specially trained in the use of different forms of radiation, including x-rays, for the treatment of cancer.

Radical cystectomy: removal of the bladder.

Sphincter muscle: a specialized circular muscle that effectively cuts off the flow of urine when contracted. Men have two such sphincter mechanisms, one at the junction of the prostate and bladder and the other just below the prostate in the upper part of the urethra. The second sphincter, which wraps around the urethra, is the one that is thought to be responsible for continence in females.

Stage: a description of the geographic location of tumors in the human body. Staging tells patients and doctors about the three-dimensional location of tumors with respect to the organ of origin as well as to adjacent structures. Staging also takes into account spread to other organs or distant sites in the body. The higher the stage, the more advanced the disease process.

Superficial bladder cancer: tumors arising from the lining of the bladder that do not invade the lamina propria or muscle wall. The majority of bladder cancers are superficial, and, though these progress in only a minority of patients, they do usually recur.

Transitional cells: the specialized cells that line the interior of the upper and lower urinary tract.

Transurethral resection (TUR): a process using a specially adapted scope that has been developed to permit the surgical removal of tumor tissue from the urinary tract through the urethra without making an incision.

Trigone: the floor of the bladder, where the ureters and urethra connect to the interior of the bladder.

Tumor suppressor gene: a member of a category of genes that are thought to be active during embryonic development. These genes have normal functions during embryonic stages that are suppressed when development is complete. If these functions are somehow reactivated during adult life, uncontrolled growth can result. This growth can sometimes lead to the development of certain cancers.

Ureter: a long, delicate tube that attaches the kidney to the bladder and carries urine to the bladder.

Urethra: a muscular tube that connects the bladder to the outside of the body and controls the flow of urine from the bladder. The urethra is surrounded by sphincter muscles that help control urine flow.

Urostomy: a form of reconstruction with a stoma to convey urine to the outside of the body.

Vesical: the medical term used for the bladder or to describe anything having to do with the bladder.

Page numbers in bold/italic refer to figures and tables.

Library of Congress Cataloging-in-Publication Data

Schoenberg, Mark P.
The guide to living with bladder cancer / Mark P. Schoenberg
and the faculty and staff of the Johns Hopkins Genitourinary
Oncology Group.
    p.   cm.—(A Johns Hopkins Press health book)
Includes index.
ISBN 0-8018-6405-4—ISBN 0-8010-6406-2 (pbk.)
1. Bladder—Cancer—Popular works. I. Title. II. Series.
RC280.B5 S34 2000
616.99'462—dc21   00-000271